For two or three couples in every hundred, artificial insemination with donor semen (AID) offers an alternative to a childless marriage. Recent public discussion of AID has concentrated on its availability, for example through commercial sperm banks, and its provision in extreme circumstances, for example to single women and lesbian couples. These 'fringe' cases, whilst important, have tended to divert attention from the much-needed more general discussion of the social consequences of AID in the community. The simple fact is that any understanding of the political effects and social implications of AID has until recently been limited by a lack of research evidence.

Dr Snowden and Professor Mitchell have used information relating to more than 1000 cases where artificial insemination was requested, and which have resulted in the birth of over 400 AID babies. This book explores the reality of those experiences of AID and provides an insight into the social aspects of a procedure which, if widely adopted, may have a profound effect on family life in the future.

The Artificial Family is written in a straightforward manner for a general readership. It avoids as far as possible technical jargon and aims to stimulate serious discussion of an important topic. It provides a concise and intelligible guide to the history, procedure, effects and implications of AID. It considers in turn the roles of the couple, the donor and the AID specialist; it examines the interests of the child and the effects on the wider family, particularly grandparents and in-laws. It discusses the issue of secrecy and the contradictions of the present legal situation; and it explores the question of AID provision to individuals and couples who do not constitute a 'normal' family and the commercialisation of AID through sperm banks and home AID kits. A section in the final chapter of the book considers the relationship between AID and other recent research activities, particularly embryo transfer – the test-tube baby of the news media – and the eugenics debate.

Dedicated to
MARGARET JACKSON
pioneer of family planning

whose interest in and concern
for childless couples has inspired
the writing of this book

The Artificial Family

ROBERT SNOWDEN has a long-standing research interest in the problems of family planning provision. He is Deputy Chairman of the U.K. Family Planning Association, a consultant to the International Planned Parenthood Federation and to the National Association of Family Planning Doctors. He is a member of the steering committee of the WHO Task Force on Service and Psycho-social Aspects of Family Planning since its inception and has just completed the co-ordination of a large cross-cultural research study concerned with the acceptability of family planning methods. He is Director of the Institute of Population Studies and Senior Lecturer in Sociology at the University of Exeter.

DUNCAN MITCHELL has taught at the Universities of Liverpool, Birmingham and Oxford and has held visiting chairs at a number of North American colleges and universities. He is Professor of Sociology, and Research Fellow in the IPS, at the University of Exeter. He has edited *The New Dictionary of Sociology* and written other books on that subject.

THE ARTIFICIAL FAMILY

A CONSIDERATION OF ARTIFICIAL INSEMINATION BY DONOR

R. SNOWDEN AND G.D. MITCHELL

Institute of Population Studies, University of Exeter

COUNTERPOINT

London
UNWIN PAPERBACKS
Boston   Sydney

First published in Great Britain by George Allen & Unwin 1981
First published by Unwin Paperbacks 1983

UNWIN® PAPERBACKS
40 Museum Street, London WC1A 1LU, UK

Unwin Paperbacks,
Park Lane, Hemel Hempstead, Herts HP2 4TE, UK

Allen & Unwin Inc.,
9 Winchester Terrace, Winchester, Mass 01890, USA

George Allen & Unwin Australia Pty Ltd,
8 Napier Street, North Sydney, NSW 2060, Australia

British Library Cataloguing in Publication Data

Snowden, Robert
  The artificial family.
1. Artificial insemination, Human—Social aspects
I. Title   II. Mitchell, G. Duncan
363.9'6   RG134
ISBN 0-04-1760026

Library of Congress Cataloging in Publication Data

Snowden, R. (Robert)
  The artificial family.
Bibliography: p.
Includes index.
1. Artificial insemination, Human—Social aspects.
I. Mitchell, G. Duncan (Geoffrey Duncan)   II. Title.
HQ761.S64   1983   363.9'6   82-23706
ISBN 0-04-176002-6 (pbk.)

Set in 11 on 13 point Garamond by
Bedford Typesetters Ltd,
and printed in Great Britain
by Guernsey Press Co. Ltd, Guernsey, Channel Islands

Contents

Preface

We all think we are knowledgeable about the family; it is a ubiquitous institution; no known society is without it; nearly all of us have had long experience of it; and yet the fact is that we know very little about the family. Indeed, it is difficult to define, it changes over time, it is perceived differently by its various members at different stages in their development, and its boundaries are constantly shifting. Thus when we come to look at the family created by means of artificial insemination by donor (AID) all these facts crowd in on us with the effect that we approach our task of discussing the subject with some hesitation.

Those like ourselves who have reflected professionally on the structures of society and the springs of human action, within psychological and sociological traditions of thought, bring to the task certain tools of the trade, but we, like our readers, have inherited values and attitudes from our own familial experiences and to be totally detached from their influence is impossible. It ill behoves us therefore to be dogmatic or to portray great certainty about the issues presented by AID. Why then have we written this book?

We wish to be explicit in this matter because in our discussion of the AID family we aver that all is not well with current practice. We are aware that to write such a book as this is to give the subject more publicity than it would otherwise have, and some would say this is unwise. But though to maintain silence may be thought advisable, to say nothing would be dishonest. An airing of the subject, if responsibly and sensitively undertaken, may be both cautionary and constructive. In the light of recent publicity and the greater extent of AID use, we believe a point has been reached where informed discussion on the subject is timely.

In this book we deal with a fundamental issue of which AID is just one manifestation; this is the problem of how we are to relate the freedom of the individual to do as he or she pleases to the welfare of society generally. This is a perennial problem and one which we cannot ignore. If there is a lesson to be learned from the history of the past two centuries it has surely been that we cannot, without serious consequences, let people do just as they like. Having said this it has to be admitted that there are few who would not subscribe to the view that as little control by the state as is possible is desirable.

We believe that the relationship of the family to the society of which it is a part needs to be explored and above all we believe that bio-technological advances demand further thought about the implications of their use. It is to this task we have addressed ourselves. Yet in doing so we are anxious to make it clear that we do not offer solutions. The social sciences have for too long been afflicted on the one hand by those who underestimate their value, saying that they merely describe the trivial in great detail and with intolerable jargon, and on the other hand by those who expect too much from them. What we endeavour to do is to raise the issues as we see them, to provide some data for informed discussion, and through psychological and socio-logical analyses to shed some light on the social processes concerned, on the origins, development and dilemmas dis-played by the kind of family that we have called the 'artificial family'. We do not raise these matters for the purpose of contributing to sensational publicity either for or against AID. We direct our remarks to that educated and informed public, many of whom may in one way or another be concerned for families and especially childless families. We have very considerable sympathy for the childless couple but, whilst this personal concern for people is never to be abrogated, we see larger issues affecting those who are not childless, and we also are concerned for all children however they came into that set of relationships we call the community or society of mankind.

Institute of Population Studies   R. SNOWDEN
University of Exeter   G. D. MITCHELL

Acknowledgements

We would like to acknowledge the work of Mrs Elizabeth Snowden, a member of the staff of the Institute of Population Studies in Exeter, without whose very considerable contribution through her researches and observations this book might never have been written, and to Mrs Ann McClary and Miss Rosalind Webber for secretarial assistance. In addition we extend our thanks to all those people, mostly anonymous, whose experience we have drawn on, and also to those who very kindly were willing to be interviewed or who wrote to us or to the press. In this last instance we gratefully acknowledge permission to publish, in whole or in part, letters sent to, and published by, the *Guardian*.

R.S.
G.D.M.

1

Introduction to the Social Aspects of AID

In 1909 Addison Davis Hard published a letter in the American journal *Medical World* in which he claimed that the first human donor insemination had been performed at Jefferson Medical College, in America, in 1884. A Philadelphia merchant and his wealthy Quaker wife, ten years his junior, had sought advice about their inability to have children. After extensive examinations of the young wife had revealed no abnormality, investigation of the husband showed him to be azoospermic, that is, he was sterile. This case was discussed in the medical school with a group of students one of whom was Hard. They suggested that semen should be collected from the 'best-looking member of the class' and used to inseminate the wife. According to Hard, this was done whilst the woman was anaesthetised and neither the husband nor the wife was informed of the process. The lady conceived and reluctantly the husband was told what had happened. Fortunately the husband was pleased, but he asked that his wife should not be told. The pregnancy proceeded normally and a son was born. The surgeon in charge of the case went to his grave with his secret, but when the merchant's son was 25 years old he was visited by Hard (perhaps the 'best-looking member of the class'!) who then published the news of this bold experiment.

In the ensuing controversy to which this publication gave rise it was revealed that Sims (another Jefferson graduate) had earlier performed artificial insemination on several women but in each case using the semen from the husband. He had, he claimed, performed a total of fifty-five uterine injections of husbands' semen and had achieved a conception rate of about 5 per cent. Nevertheless, the case of the Philadelphian businessman and his wife is the first recorded instance of artificial insemination by donor (AID) in humans.

In the ensuing uproar recriminations were heaped on the now-dead surgeon who had performed the AID, the sterile husband, the unknown donor and the medical school where it all took place. Some people who wished to defend the surgeon claimed that Hard was playing a hoax and that the events described did not take place, one even going so far as to argue that as the surgeon was a gentleman it would have been uncharacteristic for him to have behaved in the way Hard had claimed he did. In replying to the storm of controversy he had produced, Hard admitted that he had added personal comments to his account in order 'to set men thinking' but that his statement was founded on truth.

Some people argued in favour, pointing out the real needs of the involuntary childless, others appealed to sensibility pointing out the utter repugnance of AID. The eugenists were quickly on the scene and in the process divided the medical profession by their claims that the improvement of the genetic stock of America was now possible. Lawyers, moralists, theologians, medical practitioners, almost everyone joined in the debate for a short time in 1909.

The issues debated in 1909 are very little nearer resolution in 1980 than they were then. The one major difference is that AID is now practised much more widely. The conflict of how to satisfy the needs of individuals, whilst at the same time maintaining the integrity of social organisation, is one that will be debated for years to come. Indeed, the issues of genetic manipulation, the woman's right to choose and the maintenance of family life, are issues which will continue to have their protagonists and antagonists for as long as the need for social organisation endures. What will doubtless change is the social climate in which these debates will take place.

The possibility of artificial human insemination began to be discussed more seriously in this country in the 1930s as advancing medical knowledge showed that in a considerable number of childless marriages the husband was the cause of the infertility. A small group of gynaecologists used the technique during the war years for the small number of their cases where it seemed to offer the only solution, but AID remained virtually unknown to the general public until 1945 when the first comprehensive account was published in the *British Medical Journal*, provoking a considerable amount of discussion in the press and in Parliament. At the end of that year the then Archbishop of Canterbury set up a commission to inquire into the development of the practice. The report was strongly critical of AID and recommended that the practice should be made a criminal offence. Following further debates in Parliament, the Feversham Committee was appointed and its report, published in 1960, also concluded that AID was undesirable. Nevertheless, AID continued to be practised on a small scale by a few infertility specialists, and as infertile couples became more aware of this possible solution to their problems the demand for AID, whilst still remaining small, steadily increased.

The climate of public opinion on questions of sexual behaviour has undergone a considerable change and AID, though still a controversial subject, is now looked upon with less reluctance by both the medical profession and the general public. In 1970, following an increasing number of requests for information about AID, the British Medical Association appointed a panel of inquiry under the chairmanship of Sir John Peel and its report, published in 1973, was more favourable.

The procedure of artificial insemination by donor is a simple one. Semen is collected by the donor masturbating into a container which is delivered as quickly as possible to the AI practitioner either for immediate use, or for freezing and storage. Freezing the semen is complex in that it requires semen to be mixed with a cryoprotective medium containing precise amounts of glycerol, egg yolk, fructose and dilute sodium citrate. The mixing process is very carefully undertaken, the resulting mixture being divided into a number of ampoules which, after labelling, are stored in liquid nitrogen. A careful procedure is also followed in thawing the frozen semen when it is required for use. Insemination using fresh or previously frozen semen is undertaken at what is considered the optimal time in the women's menstrual cycle; that is, near the time of ovulation. This is usually ascertained by asking the women concerned to keep an accurate menstrual calendar and basal body temperature record. Using a simple plastic syringe a small amount of semen is deposited high in the vagina near the cervix or sometimes directly into the cervical canal.

It is estimated that approximately 10 per cent of marriages are infertile, and that the husband's infertility is responsible in about one-third of these couples. This indicates an incidence of about 16,000 marriages a year which will be infertile because of the husband. The Peel Report estimated that some 10 per cent of these couples (1,600) may consider AID at sometime during their marriage. AID may also provide a means of producing a healthy family for those couples where the husband suffers from a hereditary disease. Now that a genetic counselling service is offered by the national health service, it is possible for more couples to avoid the birth of an abnormal child and it is likely that some of these couples will wish to avail themselves of AID. Couples who are unable to enlarge their families because of rhesus factor incompatibility may also make recourse to AID. Another source of AID request is from those in second marriages where the husband has previously undergone voluntary sterilisation. During the past decade the demand for AID has been accelerated by the fall in availability of babies for adoption. Despite the increasing demand for, and acceptance of AID, there is still very little known about the consequences of the procedure. This is, no doubt, mainly due to the atmosphere of secrecy which has always surrounded the practice.

Although AID is not in itself an illegal practice, it leads to a situation where the legal position is far from clear. As the law stands, an AID child is illegitimate and the birth registration entry for such a child should either have the name of the donor, the words 'father not known', or a blank space left where the father's name should be recorded. But almost invariably a husband enters his own name as the father of the child and in doing so he is in contravention of the Registration Act of 1965, unless he is under the impression (rightly or wrongly) that there is a genuine possibility he may be the father. It is partly for this reason that couples undergoing AID are often advised not to abstain from sexual intercourse during the period of artificial insemination. No court in this country has, so far, considered the legitimacy of a child believed to be the product of AID and, moreover, it is thought that any court would presume a child born within a marriage to be the child of the husband and wife unless evidence to the contrary was produced. However, among those seeking AID almost all do so because of the known sterility of the husband. It would seem that in order to deal with the legal difficulties of legitimising the AID child's status, the child's parents, that is, the AID mother and her husband, have embarked on a subterfuge leading in most cases to illegal behaviour. To confer legitimate status on AID children might resolve the legal confusion but our reflections on such a change indicate that there are complexities which may lead to even greater legal, and social, confusions, for it is not only married couples or even heterosexual couples who seek AID. Nevertheless, members of the legal profession are currently considering the implications of conferring legitimate status on AID children within the whole context of the categories of legal status for children who are brought up as members of a family.

One possible solution is for the AID couple, the mother and her husband, to adopt the AID child, but this course of action merely adds to the confusion. The adoption procedures to be followed would appear absurd in such a case and, perhaps more important for the couple, there would be in existence a birth certificate declaring their adoption of the child.

Even the donor does not escape from this legal uncertainty, for it has been suggested that if the identity of a donor becomes known, he could be held responsible for the maintenance of the child or children he has helped to create and on his death his estate could be divided between the offspring he has, perhaps unknowingly, produced. It is interesting to note in this connection that legal advisers to those providing an AID service suggest that consent forms relating to AID provision should be signed by the donor as well as by the couple concerned.

Attempts have been made in other countries to resolve the legal dilemmas associated with AID but no consistent pattern has emerged. Olive Stone, writing in 1973, pointed out that in Switzerland AID is illegal, it being held to be incompatible with marriage, and a child born by AID can be disowned. In France the AID child is held to be legitimate unless an application is made by a woman's husband against affiliation, but such a denial must be made within six months of the child's birth. Portuguese law explicitly declares AID to be insufficient by itself in a dispute about affiliation. In the USA some states, for example, California, Georgia and Oklahoma, have declared AID to be legal and children to be the legitimate offspring of the mother and her husband providing he has given written consent. But Indiana, Minnesota, New York, Virginia and Wisconsin have rejected proposals to legalise AID. In Poland there is no legal notion of legitimacy; a child born within a family is held to be the child of both parents unless within six months the man denies he is the parent.

The problem surrounding the legal situation is that it induces deception and illegality in an attempt to circumvent the implications of its enforcement. This deception is often not discouraged by those acting as advisers to the AID couple. Indeed some would say that the deception is being supported and encouraged by many of these advisers who are also those providing the AID service. Falsification of records is taking place and to ignore this fact is to be party to a deceit in relation to the AID child and to society as a whole. Perhaps we should spend our energies in dealing constructively with the difficulties presented by AID rather than in trying to find ways of maintaining secrecy and the subterfuge this entails.

Merely changing the law will have little effect on the real issues surrounding AID, for the AID process is not just a legal issue. Of far more importance are the social implications of the practice. The difficulties in openly stating that a child born to a wife is also not her husband's are of such a psychological and social depth that they act as powerful incentives for the mother's husband to declare he is the AID child's father. It is hardly surprising that what evidence there is points to this being an almost universal practice.

Since the first public debates about the practice of artificial insemination by donor there have been repeated calls for assessment of the psychological and social effects of the practice. These are usually seen as affecting the quality of the relationships within the family. But the social consequences of AID are far wider than those related directly to the AID family itself – the mother, her husband, the AID child and possibly other children of the couple. In this chapter and those which follow an examination is to be made of the social and personal issues involved from two different but overlapping points of view: first, the effect upon the members of the family directly involved and those associated with them in the AID process, and secondly, the way in which the AID family as a unit is related to other close relatives, more distant relatives, friends and neighbours. How members of the AID family view themselves and each other will be affected very strongly by how they believe their relatives and friends would react to their situation. Why individuals see themselves and the others in the way they do may be related more to the influence of the wider group than we often recognise.

There are usually four people directly concerned in the AID process. These are the mother, her husband, the donor and the AI practitioner. There may be others, the family doctor, a close friend or relative, for example, but these four can be said to be the central figures participating in the actual process of producing a child by AID. It is also true to say that the husband is the only one of these four who does not necessarily have to play an active part. He is usually seen as a bystander who may be actively providing encouragement and support during the process but his role is not an essential one for the successful production of an AID child. The result of the collaboration between the mother, the donor and the AI practitioner, if success has been achieved, is the AID child. The AID child has not been listed as a participant in the AID process for the obvious reason that being the product of the process the child is not a participant in the careful planning, the detailed discussions and the inconvenient and sometimes embarrassing procedures that have to be followed in getting sperm from a healthy donor united with an ovum of a healthy woman who desires to be a mother.

By examining the relationships between those directly engaged in the creation of the AID family in some detail, it may be possible to identify those issues which act as a source of stress or uncertainty for the AID family. Through this process it is hoped that assistance and advice can be more effectively given to those contemplating the AID procedure as a means of resolving their own infertility problems. Information has been obtained through discussion with AID parents, donors and practitioners, through detailed correspondence, and a review of published information. It has not been possible to interview an AID child but correspondence has been received from some who have been informed of their AID status. Correspondence and discussions were also entered into following an airing of the subject in a national newspaper. The authors have taken special care to avoid the possibility of identification of any person providing comment or information but the desire to discuss the subject by those involved has been very obvious.

Any examination of human relationships can become very complex, especially when such relationships are based on thoughts and feelings about oneself, about others in the relationships and perhaps even more important how one thinks others think of oneself. The mother in the AID family not only has thoughts and feelings about herself as a mother, but also thoughts and feelings about her husband who in this instance is deficient in his ability to provide her with a child. But for confidence, trust and mutual affection to persist, which in turn maintain a stable marital relationship, this mother will also be responding to what she thinks her husband thinks of her. For some members of the AID family this must be more obvious than for others, but nevertheless it does affect all members of the family to some degree. Some husbands whose wives have had a baby by means of semen donated by another male outside the marital relationship have not found it easy to come to terms with their own inadequacy in this respect. The resolution of this issue appears to be very heavily dependent on what the husband believes his wife (the mother of the AID child) thinks of him.

Because of the high level of confidentiality and secrecy surrounding the AID process it is difficult to discover the manner in which people perceive the AID family, and the way in which members of the AID family believe others to perceive them. What can be said is that the secrecy, and the willingness to withstand the ensuing stress of maintaining it, indicate that a belief is held by AID couples that the attitudes towards them would be negative ones. Generally it would appear that the perceptions we have of the way others think or feel about us directly or about members of our families are powerful determinants of our self-image. It follows that if this is the case in a normal family it must surely affect the 'artificial family' much more. Moreover, whilst it may be supposed that secrecy is observed for the sake of the child, a closer examination reveals a much more complex situation. Although the issue of secrecy is considered much more fully in Chapter 5 we have introduced it here to indicate the levels at which the perception of a relationship may be viewed. Each of the four areas of perception (self-perception, perception of spouse, perception of how spouse feels about self, perception of how other relatives, friends, neighbours and acquaintances feel about self) are all interrelated and serve to create the feelings we all of us have about ourselves. These feelings need to be expressed in some way, and this usually takes the form of behaviour of some kind. Our perception of ourselves as mother, father, male, female, doctor, and so on, is translated into a form of behaviour which we believe represents how such a person would behave. We call each of these a 'role' and we all play many roles in our social and professional lives. In normal circumstances these roles are learned from those around us as we grow up. There is usually a common understanding of what constitutes a particular role so that when acting out that role it can be recognised by those around us. There are certain expectations held about what makes up a particular role. For example, in Western cultures the role of father usually implies that a man has children that are biologically his offspring. In those cases where a biological relationship is absent exceptions to the rule are usually made so that the father role may be undertaken without too much disturbance. This is what occurs when an adopted child is introduced into a family – the father plays a father role with the understanding that this is socially permissible. Indeed, when such roles become formalised they exist as part of our legal system. The law brings with it formal rights, duties and obligations which the society at large enforces by a variety of means. But what if the socially defined role of fatherhood is being broken *without* the knowledge of society at large? Can a man become a *father* of a child that is not his own offspring and is not a child which has been placed in his care by due process of the law as an adopted or foster child? At what point does a selected male cease being described as a guardian and become a father? Can an uncle to a child also become a father to the same child simply by acting out a father role?

When we speak of fatherhood, whether in the biological or psychological sense or a hazy combination of them both, we are, of course, referring to two of the four principal actors in this drama of life – the husband and the donor. The use of the word 'husband' rather than 'father' is deliberate and reflects the lack of a word to describe adequately the difference in the roles of these two men. This confusion is described to demonstrate the point that the terms 'mother' and 'father' contain within them assumptions that most of us take for granted and seldom examine. When the AID child is considered these assumptions require examination for it is in the attempts to resolve the complexities underlying them that the behaviour of AID parents can best be understood. The topic of paternity will figure again and again in the present discussion of AID; indeed it is our contention that any consideration of the social effects of AID rests squarely on the issue of paternity.

The role of the mother in the AID family is less ambiguous. The AID mother usually provides a combination of biological, social and psychological support to the child in a way that her husband cannot. She conceives, carries and gives birth to the child; a child she has taken on trust and knowing very little about the other half of the germ cells which with her own have created 'her' child. In some ways the mother has more difficulty than the other three engaged in the AID process. It is she who is biologically able to have a child and yet has to go through often embarrassing interviews, examinations and procedures in order to become pregnant. She has to provide support for her husband and hide a secret she would often like to share. But also she has an advantage over her husband in that she knows the child she has conceived is *her* child even if not her husband's.

The AI practitioner is usually a member of the medical profession but not necessarily so. The insemination procedure is not technically difficult to carry out – in fact some AID parents are known to have done this for themselves. The timing of the procedure in the menstrual cycle may need some care but even this can be accomplished without recourse to a doctor. On inquiry at a chemist's shop in London for an insemination syringe, the answer was given to one researcher – 'any syringe-like instrument will do'. Skill is required in freezing and unfreezing sperm stored in liquid nitrogen but this assumes that storage is necessary. The use of fresh semen is not uncommon and used to be even more common than it is today. If fresh semen is available and a suitable syringe is bought from a chemist's shop, anyone can do it. We shall be discussing the implications surrounding the introduction of 'home insemination kits' in the USA, but suffice it to say here that if the procedure is as simple as some say it is, why then does one need a medical qualification to administer an AID service? The answer to this question probably has more to do with the need for discretion than the need for technical expertise.

The AI practitioner is acting as a broker bringing together semen and the woman who desires that semen. The AI practitioner's role is to enable this to take place in an atmosphere of support and professionalism that removes the suspicion of uncertainty and exposure. It is the *professional status* of the doctor rather than his technical competence that is required here. This status allows what could be an embarrassing inquiry to be made or an insulting request to be avoided. An inquiry about artificial insemination is often embarrassing and assurances of the cause of infertility will have to be obtained. The medical profession would normally, and competently, be involved in such an assessment. The request for sperm might be regarded as insulting by potential donors unless they felt that the request was being made by or through a person of high professional standing. A doctor seeking such help is usually listened to and many donors respond to such a request without hesitation.

It is not only the professional status of the doctor that is important but also the understanding by those seeking help of what this professionalism means in practice. Those outside the medical profession have generally accepted that those in the profession subscribe to tenets of confidentiality and integrity at a very high level. They expect that their own situation concerning infertility and the necessary arrangements for finding a suitable donor will be dealt with in confidence and without the knowledge even of other members of the profession.

These, then, are the four principal persons involved in the AID procedure. Each has his or her own needs or a desire to help. Apart from the husband and wife, they do not know each other very well – if at all. Yet they come together to perform a task that is not particularly difficult to undertake but which has probably one of the most important outcomes imaginable – the creation of a child.

Figure 1.1 indicates that between the five people directly concerned (now including the AID child) there are ten relationships each consisting of two people (mother/husband; mother/donor; mother/AI practitioner; husband/donor;

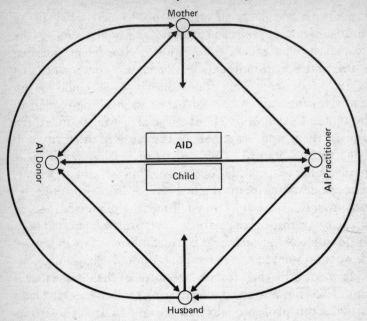

Figure 1.1 *Those involved in the creation of an AID child*

husband/AI practitioner; donor/AI practitioner; mother/ child; husband/child; donor/child; AI practitioner/ child) These provide five primary perceptual positions relating to how each views him or herself in the AID process. A further twenty secondary perceptual positions are present when one considers how each views the other four people involved. If one is to assess what each believes the others think of him or her yet another twenty tertiary perceptual positions may be discerned. Among these five people a total of forty-five perceptual positions could be examined. Some, but not all, of these are examined in the chapters which follow. A selection of the available material has been made to avoid repetition but in some cases there is little to be gleaned from the literature or from information received from AID families.

2

The AID Couple

The first question which arises when considering the AID process concerns the means by which a husband and wife reach the decision to seek information and help about gaining a child by AID. In this book we are concerned with the AID family which is created, rather than with all those who may at one time or another seek information about AID. The information we have collected to date suggests that those who reach the stage of actually having an AID child are a relatively small proportion of those who actively consider it as a means of dealing with their childlessness. In examining the relationship between the AID mother and her husband there are a number of issues to be studied. These relate to the mother herself, her husband as an individual, their interaction and the criteria which led them to seek, and be accepted as suitable candidates for AID.

THE DESIRE FOR A CHILD

Some authors (e.g. Rubin, 1965) have argued that it is the need to meet a biological drive or instinct which makes women desire a child whereas others (Piattelli-Palmarini, 1973) point to the pressures in our society which suggest that the state of childlessness is somehow 'unnatural' and that those who experience it are not fulfilling their role as responsible members of that society. These apparently conflicting views, the one biological and the other psychological, are difficult to separate and perhaps the efforts expended in attempting to do so are futile. Understanding the relationship between 'mind' and 'body' has defied the most advanced thinking. Instead we might agree that a more fruitful approach would be to examine the interaction of the two in relation to specific behaviour which is the result of their interaction.

The most important fact relating to the AID mother is that she is in no way deficient in her ability to bear a child of her own in the biological sense. She is a basically fit person whose impediment to achieving a child is not of her own making but present in her partner to whom she is usually deeply committed. In order to deal with the need to have a child, whether this is prompted by biological drives or social pressures, the norms by which our society regulates itself require that the person who provides the other half of the genetic make-up of the resulting child should be the husband of the mother; that is, someone with whom she has entered into the legally binding contract of marriage. In our society at the present time there are therefore two pressures being exerted on women. The first is the expectation of motherhood and the second is that such motherhood should take place within marriage and as a result of the participation of the husband in that marriage. Of course there are exceptions to these rules and our expectations are sometimes not realised, but nevertheless the normal way of behaving in these matters is to marry and produce offspring in partnership with the husband. To do otherwise is to be abnormal in some way which in turn leads to a need to justify the different form of behaviour.

AID OR ADOPTION?

There is also a more subtle distinction to be made when

considering the desire of the AID couple to have a child. Is it the desire to rear a child or the desire of the AID mother to bear a child that is the primary concern? There is much confusion about this. Many couples have reported that their request for AID was the result of not being able to find a baby for adoption. Among such couples the implication is that the desire to rear a child is more important than the desire to *bear* a child. The following three cases serve to make this point:

- Couple started to arrange for adoption but were told it would be at least a three-year wait – so requested AID.
- Couple had tried to adopt but found the list was closed.
- Couple inquired about adoption but found it would be impossible to adopt a baby and that the waiting list to adopt an older child was extremely long.

Among couples such as these the desire for a baby or child was paramount. In order to complete the family unit a child was needed. There is no suggestion of wanting to bear a child among such mothers; AID was resorted to as a second attempt at gaining a child after adoption was no longer an alternative they wished to pursue.

It is not merely the non-availability of babies for adoption that attracts the mother and her husband to AID; the type or perceived quality of the babies available for adoption is also an issue.

- This couple stated explicitly that they were afraid to adopt because they 'would not know where the baby comes from.

     'We both long for children and, although adoption is a possible answer, it seems preferable that any child we have will, at least, have a good chance of inheriting some of the many good and lovable traits of my wife.'

It would appear from such comments that the couple concerned have trust in the AI practitioner that the donor's background has been carefully checked and that the use of AID reduces uncertainty concerning the health, physique and personality of the child. This view is repeatedly argued but there is an obvious flaw in the argument for the child put up for adoption can be seen before the process of adoption is completed and therefore physical defects can be ascertained in advance. The AID option provides no such advance assessment. The view that the AID baby has a genetic structure contributed by the mother and is therefore less of a risk than one where the background of both parents is unknown is an interesting one. Even a cursory knowledge of genetics indicates that the variability of interaction between the genes of a known male and a known female is such that the possibility of prediction of personality type is unlikely. Yet the perceived reduction in uncertainty is understandable even if the contribution by the donor remains an unknown quantity to the potential AID couple. The need to bear a child to fulfil some deep-felt psychological need by the mother is not the primary concern in such cases. Rather there is a need to reduce uncertainty about the genetic background of the child to be introduced into the family.

There is yet another factor to take into account when considering the alternatives of adoption and AID. It is not just the non-availability of babies or 'suitable' babies but also the ability of the couple to be accepted as suitable parents by those responsible for placing available babies. In some cases adoption has been denied to inquiring couples. Refusal as potential adoptive parents because of the husband's or wife's age, health and even their way of life have been noted by the authors among those seeking the alternative of a child by AID. There are other cases where the adoption of a child has not been attempted because of the belief that a request would lead to refusal. These cases occur among single girls, lesbian couples and even the occasional trans-sexual person. Some couples or individuals who would not normally be accepted as suitable parents by an adoption agency nevertheless may be able to have a child by AID because of the different methods of assessment and the different criteria used in selection.

Even when the idea of adoption for whatever reason is not taken up it is by no means certain that the couple will be accepted as suitable AID parents by the AI practitioner. Selection for AID is usually based on the AI practitioner's impression of the suitability of the couple. What constitutes suitability is determined by the behaviour of the couple at interview, the views of the AI practitioner and available background information provided by the couple's family doctor. In some cases family doctors are opposed to AID for their patients and it is not unknown for their dislike to result in removal of the patient from the doctor's list. One couple had asked their GP for assistance and after an AID child had been born with multiple deformities and quickly died he wrote:

> I am not willing to take part in the treatment of this couple where the ultimate end is further AI. I have told —— how I feel about this and indeed he knew all my views before he consulted you in the first place. If he wishes he can change his registration in the NHS.

Nevertheless this couple went ahead and tried for three years for another AID child but without success.

In other cases the AID couples specifically ask that their family doctor should not be informed. The reasons usually given relate to the perceived antagonism of the family doctor to AID on personal or religious grounds, but it is not clear if this is what the AID couple genuinely perceive. It appears that the desire to keep the act of AID secret may also affect the family doctor/patient relationship and even the relationship between colleagues in the same profession.

Those being asked for advice about AID are sometimes reluctant to suggest the procedure, preferring that the couple concerned should seek the adoption of a child in the knowledge that if they do so their inadequacy as potential parents will be revealed to them. In one case a couple attended for AID after failing to be accepted by an adoption society, supposedly because of a negative report from a psychiatrist who had previously treated the wife. The couple's family doctor who knew this wrote:

> I am in some doubt as to the advisability of AID as compared with adoption. However much they may now agree, it will never alter the fact that with AID the child will always be hers and never his. In the event of future friction, which is to be expected in any marriage, this could well become a bone of contention, to the detriment of the child. I cannot help feeling with these two, that as far as a child is concerned, it would be better if they started on an equal footing and adopted a child with all the formalities involved.

This raises the issue of public accountability or social control of the procedures leading to couples becoming adoptive parents or AID parents. In the case of adoption there are stringent legal procedures in force but in the case of AID there are no such legal restrictions. The reasons for seeking an AID child may be more complex than they appear at first sight. At a time when the number of babies for adoption is declining the alternative procedure of AID for those couples where the wife is able to bear a child becomes more attractive. This is discussed very clearly by one correspondent following refusal by an adoption society resulting from the husband's history of alcoholism which he openly admitted and of which he was now cured. The husband wrote:

> our own doctor advised us to discuss the matter of AID if our efforts at adoption should fail – which they

unfortunately have. He sees no harm in this procedure although this is a monumental step to take for both of us – I suppose for the future more for me than for my wife – I think this [AID] is the answer. He is of the opinion that we should not wait much longer from the point of view of my wife's age and peace of mind.

This couple attempted to have a child by AID for two years and towards the end of that time they approached another adoption society and this time they were accepted. The wife then wrote explaining why she wished to discontinue AID:

We have been wondering if it is any good going on with the AID treatment. I have been having it now for over 15 months and it does not seem to be very successful. Now we are sure of having a baby by adoption, there does not seem to be much point in carrying on with it . . . I have never really liked the idea but at the time we thought it was the only way to have a baby. In a way I am happier for my husband that AID was not a success and that we are adopting . . .

This couple clearly desired a child and were prepared to go through considerable inconvenience and uncertainty in order to obtain one. It is interesting to note that AID was discontinued as soon as the couple were placed on the waiting list for an adopted child. There was no guarantee that a child would become quickly available and, no doubt, the couple would have been made aware of this by the adoption society concerned. The last sentence quoted above is a very telling one. The case of this couple with the statement by the wife concerning her husband's 'peace of mind' provides a typical situation found among AID parents. Both partners emphasise their part in the procedure in terms of the feelings of their spouses.

Another husband (who specifically asked that his letter

should be used to help others faced with a similar situation) expressed his own uncertainty about the alternatives to AID in the following way:

You have my unqualified support and approval in this work [AID] for a variety of reasons. The first reason is an entirely personal one: for a long time my wife and myself have desired a family. If we cannot have a child entirely of our own in every sense of these words, then we welcome the chance to have a child that is as much our own as is possible in the circumstances. We do not just want 'a child'; we do sincerely want 'our child'. Any child born to my wife into our house in the natural manner must be, both to us and all the world, 'our child'. The problems and pleasures to be experienced by us together during my wife's pregnancy, and the preparation to be made against the future needs of the child, my wife's subsequent confinement – all these are to my mind essential experiences which will make the baby 'our child'.

This leads to the second reason, which is quite simply that no adopted child, however loved and desired, can provide what I call these 'essential experiences'. I may be unusual and even called selfish but I do not feel an adopted child could enjoy quite the same high status as a child born to my wife. This is, of course, a personal view again, but to me an adopted child would fall short of being 'our child' because of the missing 'essential experiences'.

Thirdly, pursuing the adoption comparison, there is in my mind the brutal precept 'I want to know what I am getting'. In the process [AID] . . . I know I am getting the produce of my wife and guaranteed stock. In the case of an adopted child this safeguard does not exist. Even if I know the child's parents, never can I hope to have the intimate history necessary to provide such a safeguard . . . I do not like to risk the consequences of receiving a child from the 'wrong' background. Perhaps there is nothing at all in heredity but I cannot help asking this question: 'What if the child (for example an adopted, bastard child) inherits the weakness of its parents?' All very selfish maybe but again my personal reason for preferring 'our child' and saying that if we cannot have 'our child' then I doubt if I shall be willing to adopt one.

Lastly, in the process [of AID] there is nothing distasteful to me. In the past, advice was given to us which amounted to no less than adultery by my wife being counselled. This filled both of us with disgust. All fear of any such taint is entirely removed. Your proceedings are confidential in the extreme, the family will be 'ours' and no one can ever dare suggest that family to be the product of matrimonial misconduct. I have known a respectable married woman called 'bastard' to her face and have no action in defamation available because it was the truth. That cannot happen to 'our child' because the world will know it is as 'our child' and nobody else's.

There is no mention here of a biological need or maternal instinct for a child. The prime concern of this husband is to ensure that the child coming into his house is protected from any defamatory expression concerning its parentage. What is being argued here is for a socially acceptable child; a child that provides no evidence of its different conception. This cannot normally be accomplished through the introduction of a child after it has been born to another mother but it is possible to do this if the child is conceived by the wife leading to pregnancy and birth. Very naturally the husband is wanting to protect the child and is clearly concerned that some guarantee concerning its genetic stock is possible. It is interesting to notice that this husband's protection against the *charge* of illegitimacy in relation to the child is more important than the fact of illegitimacy. This correspondent was already aware that in law the AID child is classified as illegitimate as long as the mother and the donor remain unmarried. The need to deal with perceived social pressure resulting from the stigma of having an illegitimate child in his family was clearly important to this correspondent. It is not so much the presence of illegitimacy but the knowledge by others of its existence that is so worrying. The desire to be seen to be a conforming member of society can be a very powerful determinant of behaviour.

THE SOCIALLY CREATED CHILD

Nevertheless, the correspondent quoted above has a point. The social creation as opposed to the biological creation of a child has taken place and the husband and wife have participated in the planning of such a creation. In this sense there may be some justification in speaking of the AID child as 'ours'. When adopting, a couple take over the responsibility for an individual who has already been created by others. In AID the couple come to a mutual decision which results in the creation of a new human being. This new human being is then seen as a creation of *their* marriage and in this sense the term *social creation* has some justification. Løveset, a Norwegian gynaecologist, quotes one wife as saying:

An AID child is the result of the marriage betwen us two. We see the child as ours. To adopt a child would be more impersonal.

This point of view is also implicit in a letter written to an AI practitioner in this country:

obviously we are absolutely delighted – he is a super

baby . . . a lovely creation you have helped us create. We both thank you most warmly and hope you will accept us again next year when *we* would like to start another baby. (authors' emphasis)

And again:

We would like to thank you very much for your help and understanding that made this very happy event possible. We are very proud of *our* son . . . (correspondent's emphasis)

One of the most carefully considered letters written by an AID couple was sent to a number of national organisations who were considering AID during the time the Feversham Committee was collecting evidence about the subject. These anonymous writers placed emphasis on the spiritual aspect of married life and their desire to achieve a peace of mind within their own marriage.

I have, over the course of the past few years, noticed accounts of some of the comments which have been made on artificial insemination by donor. Few of those which have been publicised offer encouragement to those few of us where the husband is thus unfortunate . . . Until a year or so ago our interest was merely casual. However, after three years of marriage, it was discovered that I was congenitally sterile, though 100% normal otherwise. A doctor could not have found this other than by very special examination.

My wife and I were then faced with the most difficult decision of our lives to date. We were over 30 and could not afford to delay. The very long delay which adoption entails was undesirable on several counts, and after a very great deal of heart searching we took the decision to use AID. No one could make this decision for us but we had a very great deal of help from our doctors. This, regrettably we felt, was much more impartial than any assistance the church could have given us under the circumstances. Spiritual assistance probably, yes, but not the assistance which comes from personal experience and practical knowledge.

It is the privilege of a woman and duty, and a very large part of some women's lives, to bear children. I could not condemn my wife not to bear a child – in fact sterility might be considered equally sufficient as non-consummation as grounds for divorce.

Therefore, after a very great deal of thought we decided, together, that we would only have peace of mind if the child was part of us as far as was possible. In that decision we are, as the church decrees, one. My wife's pleasure will, therefore, be mine and we shall share the joy of having a child that is in a very large part our own.

The alternative, adoption, is to have a child wholly of two other persons and probably conceived and born out of wedlock. No fault of the child's, certainly, but it would appear all too easy these days to divest oneself of the responsibility of a child so born. As there is so great a demand for these children we feel that they should be left for the women who are unable to have a child of their own.

If we can find peace of mind, and this we believe to be peace with God, then surely the course we have taken is the right one . . . Never has the decision to 'start a family' been so carefully taken nor so much desired. Were there not the possibility of motherhood for my wife through AID I would have gone through life hateful of myself and in one respect a failure . . .

It is our own case we are putting forward and I have tried to stress the spiritual side. We are not devout worshippers but we do believe. And part of this belief is that we must each, individually, or together in the case of man and wife, arrive at our own salvation. The church cannot do this for us but it can help us, and we need help and, I sincerely believe, more understanding on this subject than the church has yet found possible – not sympathy but understanding.

Finally, having made our decision we cannot go back on it neither do we wish to do so. Naturally, we do not wish to enter into any controversy at this stage and so we must, regrettably, withhold our names . . .

Nothing has moved me sufficiently before to put my feelings in writing but I am most sincere in hoping that you will consider this letter in the spirit in which it is written.

This concept of the AID couple jointly creating a child is seen from a slightly different point of view by another mother in Løveset's Norwegian study:

I believe [my husband] is a bit jealous of me. Coming home after having had AI, he seemed somewhat strange. The idea occurred to me that he regretted and I therefore told him there could be no child if he did not take part in it. He is not unintelligent, but I persuaded him to have intercourse with me. Maybe that is why I succeeded in being pregnant after AI only once. Anyway, I made myself believe that as a kind of consolation.

The mutual decision to create socially a child of the marriage is not always as straightforward as it seems. The last sentence quoted gives a chilling reminder of the uncertainty of the situation irrespective of the high hopes for mutual support which often permeate consideration of AID at the outset.

It is generally accepted that the couple seeking AID should have come to a joint decision to do so but what underlies this joint decision can be very complex. It is not just what the wife and husband feel they want for themselves as individuals but also what they perceive as the wants of their partner. This has been clearly described by a Norwegian AID mother in Løveset's study:

> . . . but it sometimes strikes me as being a sin. Then it helps me to know that I did not do it for my own sake. I personally would prefer to adopt a child but my husband was absolutely against it. He was scared by the thought that people should know he was no good. I would gladly have taken the blame. On the other hand it was very unpleasant for me to be snubbed by my parents-in-law with whom we live, because they believed I was to blame for our childlessness.

What are perceived as the partner's wants in this situation may not be as simple as they appear. A desire to rationalise one's own feelings of guilt, the psychological pressures that being childless create and the frustration that keeping a secret engenders may have more to do with oneself than we would be prepared to admit.

THE DESIRE TO BEAR A CHILD

Where there is a powerful desire to *bear* a child rather than just rear a child, the use of AID to bring this about appears to be a very reasonable course of action. However, the desire for the AID mother to bear a child does not appear to be confined solely to the mother. Some husbands express the wish that their wives should bear a child with the stated hope that this would help their wives to experience a sense of fulfilment which they otherwise would be denied. This is put very clearly by one husband:

> I know my wife longs to bear a child and as I am unable to give her one, it is surely better her maternal instincts should be satisfied in this way.

Yet as discussed earlier the husband's desire for the wife to bear a child is not always associated with the husband's wish to see his wife's 'maternal instincts' satisfied. A child born to his wife during their own marriage will normally be considered his own provided the couple maintain their AID secret. This has an effect at two levels: first, there is the presumption concerning his own fertility and, secondly, the child would be passed as being a legitimate, natural child of that marriage. A number of letters have been received from husbands who describe their wives' desire for a child. Most of these are undeniably genuine but occasionally there is a hint of an unstated underlying motive on the part of the husband. In one case the husband was concerned about his wife's desire to bear a child and used this as a reason for his own interest in AID. This man's wife later denied she desired the child when explaining why she discontinued attending for AID. She indicated that her reason for discontinuing had a great deal to do with the fact that her husband was away from home for long periods! Perhaps what is being discussed here is not the desire for a child for its own sake but the desire for a child which acts as a link between the absent husband and his wife left at home. This link can be seen in the most positive or negative terms, depending upon the personalities of the couple concerned and upon their perceived marital relationship. Of course this desire to rear or to bear a child is not confined to the AID couple, but the very process of AID brings into sharper focus some of these issues which in other marriages are probably totally obscured or more difficult to discern.

Some authors (e.g. Ostrom, 1971) argue that some women suffer from 'baby hunger' to a degree that may lead to neurotic misuse of AID. This is not so odd as it may at first sight appear. Where a wife is determined to bear a child and argues persuasively with the AI practitioner, her request may be granted without adequate consideration of the outcome for the resulting child. However, it is worth remembering that a childless marriage can itself produce a state of conflict and stress that has to be dealt with in some way. The conflict created by the process of AID should therefore not be seen in absolute terms at the personal level but in relative terms. The personal conflict present in the AID procedure may be less acute than that present when having to cope with childlessness. Attempts have been made to discuss how the couple come to a decision about seeking AID but a couple consists of two people who each need to resolve distinctive issues in relation to themselves. While the wife bears the child, the husband has to come to terms with his own inability to fulfil his own wishes and those of his wife for a child which could truly be called their own.

THE HUSBAND

The reasons usually put forward by those inquiring into why husbands consent to AID can be classified under five headings:

(1) the need to satisfy the wife's maternal instincts for a child;
(2) fears that the marriage may break up if the wife's childlessness is not resolved;
(3) the desire for a child that is 50 per cent theirs;
(4) the desire to appear as a normal family;
(5) the desire for an heir.

Some of these reasons have already been discussed but it is interesting to discern the mixture of reasons covering virtually the whole range from genetic to psychological factors. Some argue, as in the House of Lords debates in the 1950s, that the husband is exhibiting selfish motives and that society should not pander to them because of the effect on the community as a whole, the family unit and above all on the well-being of the resulting child. But most of those who have been closely involved in the subject stress the opposite point of view. Far from being selfish, the husband has to cope in the best way he can with a sense of inadequacy; a sense of inadequacy which is known to be present by the person who knows him best – his wife. According to the Feversham Committee, this feeling of inadequacy may be made even worse when his wife bears the child. Here is a clear demonstration that an anonymous donor has succeeded where he has not.

> We find it very difficult to say with confidence whether the fact that the husband has been unable to play his part in procreation, and recourse has been had to AID, is or is not likely to have a disturbing effect on the marriage relationship. We think it must often happen that a husband on hearing that he is probably sterile feels a very great sense of inadequacy. It may well be that in many cases he feels that by consenting to AID he will be doing what he can to compensate his wife for his own failure, and if a child is born, his own sterility may cease to worry him because his wife has after all been able to bear a child. On the other hand he will realise that it was most probably no action on his part but the contribution of a donor which was the physical cause enabling his wife to overcome her childlessness. Far from putting an end to his feelings of inadequacy, the continued presence of an AID child may serve only to remind him of his failure, to which he might otherwise have become reconciled with the passage of years.
>
> (Feversham Committee, 1960, para. 125)

This comment was written just twenty years ago and there is still no resolution of this uncertainty today. A much larger number of published papers is available now than was available in 1960 but these have continued in the main to express opinion and conjecture rather than describe the experience of those who have resorted to AID. It would appear that those couples who are able to accept the situation of infertility experience a strengthened marriage relationship but where this situation has not been accepted at the personal level the result can be disastrous. If the wife resents her husband for his inability to provide her with a child; if the husband has a sense of guilt and this is reinforced by his feelings that his wife's resentment is justified; if the husband resents his wife blaming him for something over which he has no control; then the hidden combination of frustration, hate and guilt is potentially very dangerous. This was one of the arguments developed by the Archbishop of Canterbury's commission reporting in 1948; a commission which concluded that the wisest course would be to make the practice of AID a criminal offence.

THE WIFE

However, feelings of guilt are not necessarily confined to the husband. Both during and following the birth of an AID child some women have reported feelings of intense stress caused by feelings of guilt. In one study (Gerstel, 1963) four of the five women seeking subsequent psychological help are reported as having refused an anaesthetic during confinement for fear they might divulge the secret of the child's conception unconsciously. This particular study has reported the behaviour and feelings of these women from a psychoanalytic standpoint and as a consequence may be criticised by those not sharing this particular point of view. The stress associated with these feelings of guilt may result from keeping the AID secret from those surrounding the AID mother, and this during what may be considered a vulnerable time for her, but guilt does sometimes appear in a more complex form. The following is part of a letter written by an AID mother who not only feels she has been unfair to her husband but also has experienced a deep need to talk to someone about her feelings:

> I must tell you I didn't *want* to write, I wanted to live an ordinary family life and forget all the trouble I had before the children were born and the manner of their birth, etc. Can you understand that? I must tell you, too, that I have been through a great deal, one way and another during the last two or three years. . . . The trouble started, I think, because I began to think my husband had regrets about the family (although he *swears* this is not true, he says he has never regretted having the children). Also as a child I belonged to the Roman Catholic Church and although I was not a practising Catholic after my marriage, the training and teaching of that church still affected me. Well, to cut a long story short (after months and months of secret worry about my husband's feelings, etc.), I read in a newspaper that the pope had said that it was criminal to have children in this way and that anyone in Italy found using this method would be sent to prison. It was the last straw as far as I was concerned. I carried on in a sort of daze for a time, I don't know whether it was weeks or months, I let the house go to pieces, I didn't care how I looked, I felt I hated my husband for a time . . . I know it is dreadful, it was absolute hell for both of us for a time and I had no one of my own to turn to for help.

This letter was followed by others over a period of time. The husband also wrote demonstrating clear support for his wife and stating that he had no regrets about AID, 'and have never had any regrets'. This couple have clearly suffered in relation to the wife's feelings of guilt and they both regret that there was no one with whom they could talk out the problem which they shared. The story has a happy ending in that a means was found to discuss the matter with local clergy but their difficulties serve as a reminder that the AID process may act as a precipitating factor in creating long-term feelings of guilt.

Many husbands appear to believe that AID will resolve a wife's desire for a child and that once the child is born a wife will not experience further stress. Such husbands are missing the point described so vividly above that a child which is 'hers' and 'not his' may continue to create stress for the wife. Nevertheless, although the husband of the AID child's mother may not be biologically linked to his wife's child the evidence we have collected suggests that he is in no doubt that he is the child's father.

EFFECT ON MARRIAGE

Almost all published reports describing AID conclude that 'the emotional and psychological problems within marriages where AID children have been born are few' (Rubin, 1965). Indeed some go further and argue that such marriages are improved and enriched (Jackson and Richardson, 1977). It is interesting to note that most of those who publish these positive statements are AI practitioners themselves. The uncertainty about the procedure is more often expressed by those who are not actively involved in providing an AID service. It is usually left to psychiatrists or departmental committees to argue that AID leads to severe disturbance in family relationships (Gerstel, 1963) or to raise other doubts about the procedure (Feversham Committee, 1960). When considering the effect on the wife and husband both those in favour of AID and those against it stress the biased nature of the information collected by their opponents. The AI practitioner will only obtain information from 'satisfied' customers and the psychiatrist only sees those who are suffering psychological stress.

Despite the claims made by many AI practitioners that the marriages in which AID has taken place are very stable or even enriched, some do inevitably fail. In many of these failed marriages the fact that an AID child or children are present appears to be irrelevant to the failure but in others the presence of the AID child is either the ostensible cause of the failure or is used by one partner to hurt the other. There are a number of instances where, following separation or divorce, the husband continues to visit the child.

When the AID child was 4 years old, the mother wrote to say her husband had left her but that this was nothing to do with AID. Her husband was still very fond of the child and visited the child each week.

This type of continued close association with the child by the husband, after his marriage to the child's mother has failed, is not uncommon and in some cases shows a very deep attachment between the husband and the child. Some husbands even appear to have a deeper relationship with the AID child than the mother, especially where the child has gone to live with the husband after separation from the mother. One such husband indicated his feelings following an inquiry about how he was getting on:

[The AID child] sees his mother as frequently as this can be managed by her. [The child] is a wonderful child. Good health and a goodness of spirit beams out of him. My ex-wife and I are united in our love for him. He does not appear to have been scarred by the parting and I pray that this will remain the case. . . . He loves his school and works and plays very hard indeed. He is very happy and arrived at the age of 11 with a well-developed moral sense. He is well loved but has not been spoilt and has been subjected to a reasonable amount of old-fashioned discipline.

At this point the letter describes the life of the two who are clearly deeply attached to each other. It is not being reproduced for obvious reasons but the last paragraph of the long letter reads:

> I am writing of the only human being I love more than myself and it is very hard to be truly objective in describing the qualities of my son.

This very moving and sensitive letter demonstrates that the capacity for affection between adults and the children whom they care for can be very deep even when those children are known not to be one's own offspring in the biological sense. Clearly this writer's marriage failure had nothing to do with the AID process or the AID child that resulted. It could be argued that the same feelings would have been generated if the child had been an adopted child rather than an AID child; the sensitivity of the writer would suggest that this would have probably been the case, but there is no way of knowing this. Such a positive outcome of the social creation of a child, even allowing for the marital disharmony that surrounded it, tends to counter the criticisms that are often made of AID.

Unfortunately the use of the AID process or even the AID child directly, either as an object of dissention or as a weapon for attack in a failing marriage, occurs more frequently. Where the AID marriage does fail, the experience of AID is sometimes cited as evidence of the failure. This may be directly attributable to AID as a discrete subject or more commonly to a fusion of the problems of childlessness and the couple's attempts to deal with this by means of AID. One wife wrote to explain why she would be no longer attending for AID:

> I've been feeling rather miserable over deciding to give AID a trial, since not only has the identity of the donor concerned me more than I thought it would but the reception of my husband of a failure 'to deliver the

goods' was not quite as sweet as might have been thought had it occurred to me previously. Please do not assume that he has been in any way unpleasant, far from it, but there now exists that uncomfortable frame of mind caused by his attitude of 'there you are, I'm not the only one' . . .

The wife is here accusing the husband of apparently vindicating his own infertility by drawing attention to his wife's inability to conceive by AID. But the issue is a confusing one showing a great deal of uncertainty by the wife. She is clearly uncomfortable about the AID process now that she has attempted to become pregnant. It is her perception of her husband's attitude which she is using to justify her discontinuation of AID. Her very natural reference to the AI donor creates some feeling that it is just as well she did not become pregnant by AID during the attempts that were made.

In the above case there was no child, but much more serious is the situation where the child's AID status is brought into the dispute. This couple had an AID child of 5 years of age. The husband wrote:

I am writing to ask if you can advise me regarding [my child] who was born with artificial insemination. My marriage to my wife has now broken up and I can see no way for a reconciliation between us. She has always held it against me for not being able to produce children, which is very unfortunate, so in order to make her happy we both agreed to her having artificial insemination. I was so happy when [my child] was born as she was such a beautiful child and still is. Since this separation I cannot see [my child] and my solicitor is helping me regarding her welfare. The last three years my wife has repeatedly told me I am only her guardian. I love [my child] very much and have always shown a great deal of affection but the hurtful part of all this is that my wife has told her I am only her uncle which is very hurtful after nearly five years . . .

Another husband wrote at a time he was trying to save his marriage but he eventually sued for divorce.

The relationship between myself and my wife has unfortunately deteriorated. Things have been getting worse for some considerable time and I am asking her to postpone any ideas she has in the meantime about another AID pregnancy . . . As I see it, people get married and if one or other partner cannot contribute to the production of children then the fact has to be faced squarely and a decision taken. I guided her initially into the decision we took thinking that she would be satisfied with about two children notwithstanding her ambition for six. She now wants to press on for more and more children but at the same time is terribly resentful of my inability to contribute and she seems to harbour a very real grudge against me. This situation is frankly intolerable. To me it represents a great contradiction – she wants to increase her family but at the same time break down the family by inflicting considerable mental pain on her husband, the man who will assume responsibility for fatherhood. All sense of partnership is thus lost . . .

Here is another sad letter, this time from an AID mother who was involved in divorce proceedings:

he continuously avoided taking the baby and I out, but persisted in going out three or four nights a week and maintained [the child] was my responsibility . . . I know I should not have but I stated to my husband it was because [the child] was not his, he did not want to play with and love [the child] freely . . .

After the divorce this husband cut off all contact with his ex-wife and child.

Letters have also been received from solicitors acting for either the husband or the wife involved in divorce proceedings, sometimes long after the experience of AID. Inquiries about the status of the child, or children, of the marriage and even evidence of the fact of artificial insemination are sometimes sought. Clearly, in a case of divorce or separation AID may be a complicating factor, and what started out as the means for resolving a human need may sometimes end by being used to justify the breakdown of the relationship which created the need in the first place.

Looking through the very large number of letters received from AID couples, one gains the impression that there are more second marriages than one would expect amongst the correspondents. It may be that when a marriage remains childless it is more readily broken down than if there are children to consider. When a couple marry with the expectation that they will have children, the discovery that this is not possible owing to male infertility may put great stress on the marriage leading, in some cases, to the break-up of that marriage.

- Husband's first marriage ended in divorce because of his inability to father children.
- Husband found to be subfertile late in his first marriage and divorced because of this.
- Husband found to be azoospermic during first marriage which broke up because of this.

These three examples, and there are many others, are provided by those attending for AID during their second marriage. Some couples marry with prior knowledge that the husband is sterile; either the husband is already aware of some medical condition or injury which has rendered him sterile or he has been investigated during a childless first marriage.

There are two issues which these findings raise. The first concerns the effect of male as compared to female sterility on a marriage relationship where such sterility is discovered during the marriage. The second relates to the effect of prior knowledge of male sterility on the success of a marital relationship. In recent years the issue of prior knowledge of sterility has been affected by the increasing number of men who have undergone a vasectomy operation during an earlier marriage. If this marriage subsequently fails and the ex-husband remarries a request for AID is sometimes resorted to after reversal of the vasectomy operation has either failed or has been discounted as a possibility.

There is an added difficulty for the sterilised male who is marrying for the second or subsequent time. He usually already has children of his own from the previous marriage. This means that his new wife, who is capable of bearing children, may feel at a disadvantage in terms of her husband's relationships with her when compared to his previous family. Among men who re-marry and who have not had a vasectomy operation, the usual method of cementing the new relationship is by having a child or children. Once this has occurred the new wife is not at a disadvantage when compared to the previous wife who has had children by this husband. This disadvantage cannot be so resolved when the husband has embarked on a procedure which has rendered him incapable of begetting further children. A resort to AID may reduce this disadvantage especially if others coming into contact with the later marriage believe that the child, or children, born within that marriage are those of the husband and wife. A letter received from a family doctor suggests that this is an important reason for the desire of a child in a second marriage.

—— has children from that [first] marriage who frequently visit and obviously give rise to some divided loyalties on his part . . . they [the second marriage] only want one child . . . She is a very pleasant but introspective girl who I feel sure partly at any rate wants a pregnancy to cement their relationship and accentuate her role in his life.

Sometimes the secret of AID spans more than one marriage. Where a couple have a child by AID and that marriage later fails or one of the couple dies, it may happen that remarriage takes place. It is not known how the AID child is usually described to the new husband or wife but in at least one case a second husband was not informed of the AID status of his wife's child. It is not clear why there is reluctance to inform the new partner and without a detailed knowledge of the family relationships involved it is not possible to generalise on this subject. Nevertheless, keeping such information away from later partners gives some indication of the pressure to appear to have led a 'normal' life in relation to fertility.

Despite these difficulties which some couples have after recourse to AID, the most important feature for the vast majority of them is that the procedure gave them hope. This appears to be so even when AID did not produce a child. One wife gave up AID to adopt children but when writing with news of her adopted children she said:

Please don't count us as a failure, at least you gave us hope, and peace of mind, that everything humanly possible was done, and it helped us a lot to reconcile ourselves to adoption.

Having an AID child to cement or strengthen the relationship between the infertile husband and his wife may result in the desired effect where the marriage relationship is already a close and strong one, but correspondence from some couples indicates that, even when they believe they have adequately thought through the implications of introducing an AID child into their relationship, the child, nevertheless, has subsequently become an object of marital dissention. If this is so for those in the initially strong marriage relationship, the prognosis for those who are seeking such a resolution for a weak marital relationship is much less optimistic. The need for efficient counselling and selection procedures is therefore not only obvious but essential if the AID procedure is to be beneficial to those for whom it is intended.

THE SELECTION OF THE AID COUPLE

The need for counselling before AID is attempted may appear obvious but who should undertake this counselling and on what basis the selection of AID couples should rest is far from clear. Some would argue that even the suggestion of selection is a repugnant one possessing overtones of eugenic selection. Others wish to see very clear conditions rigidly applied to the practice in order to ensure the best possible opportunity for the child.

First, let us examine what has been said about the selection procedure and what criteria are usually stated as being most frequently used in deciding which couples will, or will not, receive co-operation in their search for an AID child. One criterion has already been discussed: the couple must come to a joint decision and both be agreed that AID is what they want. The difficulty in ascertaining whether or not this mutual agreement exists is hard enough but to assess what might occur in the future concerning the relationship between the partners requesting AID needs much foresight, experience and training. Reaching a decision about the possibility of AID often takes a number of years resulting from the slow realisation of infertility and delay in seeking medical assistance. The decision whether to provide AID is usually based on an interview with the person providing the AID service and reports by the couple's family doctor. Some centres employ a trained social worker to provide a counselling service but this is not general.

The AI practitioners who have published details of their work use various criteria in the selection of AID couples. Suggested criteria include:

(1) Only strongly motivated couples are considered.
(2) The husband must be sterile, or subfertile, or possess rhesus incompatibility or adverse genetic factors.
(3) The wife must be free from hereditary disease and able to care for the child.
(4) The wife must be mentally and physically able to care for the child.
(5) There should be no deeply ingrained fears or prejudices about the practice.
(6) There must be a mutual understanding between the husband and wife and an apparent potential mutual understanding between the mother and child and between the husband and child.
(7) The family environment must be 'good'.
(8) The couple must be 'childworthy'.
(9) The life expectancy of both the husband and wife should be reasonable.
(10) The desire for a child should not be merely a response to peer or parental pressure.
(11) The couple must be able to give the child suitable intellectual chances in life.

Some AI practitioners stress the need for a careful psychological assessment of AID couples – sometimes calling on those with relevant professional qualifications to provide background reports on potential AID couples. Yet when this additional professional person is not part of the medical team an obvious problem arises in that information about the AID couple is known outside the medical setting. The perceived need for confidentiality, anonymity and secrecy may deter such a request for outside professional help. Indeed, whilst recognising the need for advice in some cases from a medical social worker or the couple's GP, Ledward & Symonds (1976) believe that 'the difficulty in donor insemination programmes lies in the selection of suitable recipients and we believe that this responsibility should remain with the Obstetrician'.

Such a view is not surprising at a time when bureaucracy in the national health service means that maintenance of anonymity for the AID couple is becoming increasingly difficult. Letters are typed and records updated and filed and in a busy hospital environment the capacity of the AI practitioner to keep all relevant information to himself gets progressively harder.

The selection criteria listed above, taken from published reports, indicate the enormity of the task facing those responsible for providing the AID service. The questions which immediately come to mind relate to the means by which each of these criteria are assessed and the identification of the person or persons capable of making such an assessment. How is 'strong motivation', 'mutual understanding', 'good family environment' and being 'child-worthy' to be assessed? The AI practitioner with a great deal of medical experience to fall back on may have acquired, in the course of his professional life, a considerable understanding of people and the reasons for their behaviour but this is not the same as possessing a counselling skill. Gerstel points out that the skills the AI practitioner possesses are also not necessarily relevant to an understanding of complex marital interaction and family relationships.

Even the medical criteria such as the life expectancy of the husband are open to criticism. In the case of fertile couples desiring a child, no assessment is made of the life expectancy of the couple before the child is conceived. Why should this then take place among AID couples? A selection is taking place in which the criteria for selection are ill-defined and as a consequence are likely to be poorly assessed. Gerstel goes on to say that it is the selection and counselling of prospective AID couples that are the key issues which determine success or failure in the resulting AID family. Evidence from adoption studies has shown that the successful factors in placing children for adoption did not lie so much with the child as with the attitudes of the adoptive parents. If the quality of parenthood is so important in the case of adoption where both parents start on an equal footing in relation to the child, how much more is this quality important in the case of AID where the relationship with the child is far from equal.

Most AI practitioners who have written about their AID experience indicate that they discuss with the couple concerned the legal, psychological and religious problems which may be associated with AID but they do not say how these topics are dealt with. Unlike the Archbishop of Canterbury's commission, the Feversham Committee in 1960 did not wish to see AID branded as a criminal offence but it did suggest that the practice should not be encouraged in any official way. This uncertainty about AID was due, in part, to this delicate issue of determining whether or not the AI practitioner has the necessary skills to be given responsibility for selecting the AID couples. Since then this uncertainty has not been resolved, despite the involvement of counsellors other than the AI practitioner taking part at some (but not all) of the NHS centres currently providing an AID service. This uncertainty can only be exacerbated when the issue of providing AID to a married woman without the husband's consent or even knowledge is publicly discussed. Some have claimed that the provision of AID is justifiable if the husband does not know he is sterile, and telling him so might be 'hurtful' to him (Løveset, 1951). This type of situation is in clear contravention of what most AI practitioners claim to be a necessary condition in selecting the AID couple: the demonstration that the husband and wife are in agreement that AID should take place.

There is also one published account where this issue of secrecy between the husband and wife was taken one step further – this time it was the wife and AID mother who was being deceived. The couple concerned jointly agreed to AID but the husband privately arranged with the AI practitioner that the donor should be his (the husband's) brother. In the early days of AID this was not an uncommon practice. Writing in 1945, Barton advised that although using a brother as a donor might appear the first choice owing to genotypical resemblance, it was inadvisable as the choice 'is usually incompatible with secrecy, leading to emotional disturbances involving both husband and wife'. Even so, Barton assumed that the AID couple would be aware of the brother's involvement. In the more recent case, the wives of *both* brothers were kept in ignorance of what the brothers and the AI practitioner had arranged. The sisters-in-law were much more closely related than they realised. The AI practitioner writing about this in 1975 clearly considered that such a course of action was correct in the circumstances and that keeping the wives in ignorance of the deception was justifiable:

> In two instances where the request concerned the brother we accepted it after carefully evaluating the entire problem. In order to limit as much as possible future indiscretions, the wives both of the donor and of the receiving couple were not made aware of this decision. Considering that the result from these two particular cases is the creation of happy family relationships, we have no regrets.
>
> (Schoysman, 1975)

The selection of donors is discussed below but this particular case is presented here to demonstrate the dangers of embarking on a process of deception over which there is minimal social control. It is clear that those making the decision to keep others in ignorance are acting from what they feel are the best of motives but deception, by its very nature, has no clear boundary. Should husbands who erroneously believe their sons or daughters to be biologically related to them be told the truth? Should a wife who accepts AID be kept in ignorance that by arrangement the donor is closely related? Once deception has been introduced it becomes exceedingly difficult to control. It even has the capability of creating uncertainty and doubt where no deception is present.

In the published accounts of AID it is interesting to discern important differences in the approach to selection of couples for AID. On the one hand there is the strongly held view that the AI practitioner knows best and, on the other hand, there is the desire to present as much information as possible to the inquiring couple and then to leave it to them to decide for themselves. The difference really stems from how individual AI practitioners see their role in determining whether or not the AID child is likely to be born into a suitable family environment. It is this perceived responsibility which leads to the description of suitable AID parents as 'childworthy', and so on. One author and AI practitioner has gone so far as to suggest that 'If the couple are very simple-minded people who are unlikely to be able to give the child the intellectual chances in life that he might have under better circumstances, then the proposal has to be dropped'. (Schoysman, 1975.)

It is precisely because there is no clear definition of what such terms as 'childworthy' or 'intellectual chances' mean or how they are arrived at that the AI practitioner is open to criticism. There is another assumption within the selection procedure which is also seldom made explicit. This relates to the couples who are refused AID. There must be those who are refused AID and except for the occasional reference (e.g. Schoysman, 1975, quoted above) little is learned of the circumstances of these couples and the reasons given for their rejection.

In an attempt to avoid the difficulty of making value-judgements about who should and who should not be AID parents, some AI practitioners are very careful to leave the final decision to the couple. For example, Goldenberg and White reported in 1977 that in their AID practice they

> strongly believe that once provided with adequate information and counselling, each couple has the right to make their own choice. If the couple chooses AID, we try only to determine if they are relatively comfortable with their decision, to discuss beforehand some of the possible conflicts they may have and then to proceed as they desire.

And one gynaecologist writing about a particular request for AID included this sentence: 'I must say . . . I am not very keen on AI . . . in their case but it is not my job to act as God.'

Such statements illustrate some of the doubts surrounding the selection of AID couples and how AI practitioners (which usually means doctors) see their role in deciding who should or should not have children by means of AID. Kerr and Rogers, writing in 1975, made the point that rather than justifying the selection of AID couples those involved need to justify the withholding of an AID service from those who seek it. These AI practitioners then discuss some of their own selection criteria. For example, the husband's infertility may be associated with general illness which, in turn, may have a guarded prognosis. In such cases they do not take a rigid stance of refusing these couples, but where the husband's life is currently threatened they advise delaying AID until this medical crisis is resolved. Similarly, they believe the wife's life expectation should be reasonable. That is, they would probably *not* accept a diabetic wife or a woman older than 37. Kerr and Rogers also set out psychological criteria in an attempt to ensure that the couple have come to terms with the husband's sterility in a mature and adult fashion. They suggest interviews are best carried out by a pair of interviewers, preferably a man and a woman working as a team, and that AI practitioners should have access to specialist advice. A consultant group should jointly advise in all cases of prospective AID. Such a group should include a social worker, a psychiatrist, a lawyer and possibly a clergyman in the belief that such people would improve the accuracy of predicting the suitability of AID couples.

Clearly, much of this is very laudable. AID is not a matter to be taken lightly (any more than deciding to start any family should ever be taken lightly) but these suggestions remain as suggestions and are not part of general AID practice. In any case, one gets the feeling that suggestions of this sort are presented to reduce possible criticism of the selection procedures rather than for the stated reason of obtaining more objective methods of predicting AID success. The question of what constitutes AID success is one that creates even more uncertainty and therefore the suggestion to set up a group of experts to determine the likely success of the process would be, to say the least, a little premature. The criteria for assessing a successful AID outcome have never been clearly stated and in a society where the contentedness or happiness of individual families in the normal situation cannot be predicted, the assumption that this can be predicted in the AID family does not appear realistic. It would seem unjust and a denial of human dignity if those of us who wish for a child within marriage are required to seek clearance from such a group as Kerr and Rogers suggest. Why then should the AID couple, who already have difficulties enough, be required to do so?

It would appear that there is some justification in arguing that the selection of AID parents may be much more of a problem than the selection of donors as some AI practitioners have suggested. But perhaps this belief is due to the relationship the AI practitioner has with the AID couple and with the donor. In the first case, the couple seek the AI practitioner whereas in the second it is the donor who is sought by the AI practitioner.

3

The Donor

There are two areas of major interest when considering the person who donates the semen in the AID process. The first concerns the identity of the donor and his selection, and the second concerns his perceived relationships with the others directly involved – the couple, the AI practitioner and the child. The major problem when attempting to study the role of the donor is caused by his anonymity. This means that not only is his identity not generally known but also the numbers of donors used cannot be estimated. No details are recorded on a national basis and it has proved to be impossible to obtain such information from those providing the AID service. The use of the word 'stranger' to describe the donor by French AI practitioners, unintentionally perhaps, makes this point very well.

The reason for this lack of information is, of course, due to the secrecy and confidentiality which surrounds AID. Donors are not usually known even to each other and it is only in rare circumstances that a donor has made public his involvement in a particular case. One recent example of this is the doctor who donated his own semen using AID procedures to provide a child for a woman who was in a homosexual relationship and who, with her partner, wished to have a child of 'their own'. This case was reported in the national press and discussions took place in both the medical and legal professions concerning the doctor's action. But publicity at this personal level is very rare. Almost all aspects of AID work are undertaken quietly and without publicity – to do otherwise would create serious stress for the majority of childless couples who have turned to AID for help and would, AI practitioners believe, destroy the AID service they have so carefully built up.

The perceived need for anonymity is different for the donor than for the AID couple. The donor has not attended the AI practitioner as a patient requiring treatment in the way the AID couple have. To divulge information about the AID couple would clearly be seen as a breach of medical *confidentiality* in the traditional form. This is not so obvious when considering the donor where the need for confidentiality is indirect in that it is a throw-over from the relationship with the couple. It is for this reason that the donor must remain *anonymous*. The difference between these words 'confidential' and 'anonymous' is important for they imply different reasons and even mechanisms for maintaining a secret which others are not normally allowed to share. There is a difference in the underlying motives or reasons for the secrecy. Medical confidentiality is not the same thing as anonymity and to justify one in terms of the other will lead to possible misunderstanding of the ethical considerations on which particular words are based. The AID couple are treated in confidence whereas the donor must remain anonymous. This distinction has an important bearing on any consideration of the future regulation of AID provision. How to maintain confidentiality whilst at the same time dealing with the problems of anonymity is reminiscent of the debates which preceded the more open approach which now allows an adopted child to make inquiries about his or her biological origins.

SELECTION OF DONORS

There has been no systematic study of AID donors but this

does not mean that no information exists about them. Papers published by AI practitioners have often indicated who they recommend as donors and how they are selected. The most popular group from which donors are recruited appears to be medical students. Fertile husbands of patients who have previously been treated by the doctor and colleagues and friends of the AI practitioner may sometimes be used.

It is of interest to compare the characteristics of the chosen donors with the list of recommended characteristics appearing in the published literature and written by AI practitioners in recent years. The donor should possess a combination of such traits as:

(1) good health;
(2) intelligence;
(3) good and stable personality;
(4) proven fertility (some believe at least two healthy children is the minimum);
(5) pleasing personality;
(6) free from cultural taboos;
(7) right calibre;
(8) right ethics;
(9) happily married;
(10) own wife has no history of repeated abortion;
(11) no history of congenital or mental disease in own family;
(12) not known to couple (or more specifically the mother);
(13) 'better' educated;
(14) personally known to the AI practitioner;
(15) not liable to suffer guilt or obsessional feelings;
(16) close physical resemblance to husband;
(17) likelihood of moving away from area;
(18) accessibility and availability;
(19) willing to give semen after period of sexual abstinence.

Most AID couples would probably feel that these criteria for the selection of donors give considerable comfort. The absence of such criteria as social background, ethnic origin, religious affiliation and nationality may concern some couples but such concern is usually explained away by pointing out that they are included by implication (e.g. intelligence, physical resemblance, stable personality, etc.) and that to make them explicit might cause unnecessary offence. No one actually says that donors should be English and middle class but the implication is nevertheless present. What is of most interest here is how it is possible to assess the listed criteria and how these relate to the donors most frequently used – medical students.

Because of the difficulty of obtaining donors, the AI practitioner's freedom of choice in their selection is not as wide as at first it might appear. Who becomes a donor is determined as much by his availability as by any other criterion. What appears to determine whether or not the donor is an unmarried medical student or a non-medical married man apparently has more to do with the accidents of availability than it is a result of careful planning. Where an AID service is provided in a teaching hospital almost all the donors are medical students, whereas if the service is being offered outside the hospital environment the donors tend to be married men from a variety of backgrounds.

At this stage no criticism is being made of who becomes a donor in these different settings. Indeed, each group (the medical and the non-medical) can be justified without undue difficulty. What is of interest is the conflicting criteria used when the two groups are compared and when what appears to be an attempt to rationalise the choice is made by reference to a set of criteria which has really been dictated by expediency. Who becomes an AI donor is, we believe, a matter of social concern and if a criterion for selection in one situation appears as a criterion for non-selection in another, then questions must be raised concerning the validity of that criterion.

When discussing the selection of donors, what is really

being discussed in most cases is the relationship between the donor and the AI practitioner. Who the AI practitioner seeks and selects as a donor has obvious eugenic implications. The selection of donors in combination with the selection of suitable AI couples places a great responsibility on the AI practitioner: a responsibility which, because of the principles of confidentiality and anonymity, is being discharged without external regulation of any kind.

The implications of eugenic control are recognised by most AI practitioners but often in a limited way. In discussion of this topic (e.g. McClaren, 1973) it is usually argued that the possibility of eugenic interference is reduced if the offspring of a specific donor are strictly limited in numbers. If there are few offspring, the chances of half-brothers and half-sisters subsequently meeting, falling in love and having children of their own, in ignorance of their true relationship, would be much less likely to occur. Again, if there are harmful recessive genes present in the donor's sperm, these would not be spread disproportionately within the general population if the offspring of the donor concerned are few in number. The number of four, five, or six offspring from each donor has been suggested but there is no way of knowing if the number of offspring is, in fact, so limited. 'Good' donors are not easy to find and having found one the thought of denying a childless couple (who may reside a long distance away) simply because an available donor has been too successful may appear unreasonable.

The desire to limit the offspring is one of the reasons given why medical students are considered to be a better choice of donor than married men. Medical students are unlikely to remain in the area where they have been recruited. Married men living within the local community, at least local in terms of where the AID service is provided, may remain for decades and as a result could, in theory at least, be used as donors many times. The dangers here are twofold: first, the number of offspring may be more than the few recommended and, secondly, the problems of donor anonymity may be more difficult to sustain over time. Donors as well as AID mothers often need to tell someone about their experience.

It is not just the biological hazards of subsequent inbreeding that need to be considered if large numbers of donor offspring are present. In fact, it could be argued that the fears being expressed at this level are of little significance in the present situation. The dangers of half-brothers and half-sisters, unknowingly related to each other, having children of their own are probably greater through the occurrence of adultery in most communities in our society than through the process of AID. Of far more importance are the social consequences relating to the selection of donors. It may be that the number of offspring to each donor can be kept to a limited number but if the majority of donors were tall, blond, blue-eyed and Anglo-Saxon, the *overall* eugenic effect of selection would be obvious. If male medical students are known to possess particular social and psychological characteristics which are in some way distinctive, and if donors are being deliberately selected from this group, then eugenic selection is taking place in a planned way. In most cases attempts are made to match the donor and the sterile husband, but this matching is usually confined to such physical features as colour of eyes, colour of hair and height. In this sense, the hypothetical example of the tall, blond Anglo-Saxon donor is weak, but what of 'personality', 'stability', and 'intelligence' described as important in the list of recommended characteristics presented earlier? In addition, what of creativity, the need to achieve, and what some have called 'an innate moral sense'? If donors tend to be selected from among those who possess (or lack) one or more of these traits, then eugenic selection is taking place and should be discussed.

It is often asserted that with medical students as donors, at least one can be sure that the 'right sort' has been selected. An acceptable level of intelligence, education and a character of the 'right calibre' is assumed among those seeking entry into the medical profession. The assumption that medical students are 'not liable to suffer guilt or obsessional feelings' or that they are 'free from cultural taboos' nevertheless leaves one with the feeling that the whole issue of donor selection needs radical reappraisal. How the criteria for donor selection are to be assessed and who should be responsible for such selection and assessment remains an issue requiring urgent consideration.

Another issue concerning the use of medical students as donors is the possibility that these young men are not making a choice about donating semen on the same basis as other men outside the medical profession. Perhaps young medical students who are entering a profession with much idealism about helping others, and who are asked by their seniors and teachers to help in this particular way, may later regret their action when they are more mature and less dependent upon those who are responsible for their initial training. The convenient availability of medical students within the hospital environment is a very powerful determinant of their involvement in the AID procedure. It would be of interest to inquire if more senior hospital medical staff (e.g. housemen, registrars and consultants) are also recruited in proportionate numbers. If not, what are the underlying reasons for this discrimination?

This issue of availability is also a factor in the consideration of the use of frozen or fresh semen. When frozen semen is used there is a readily available supply of semen for a busy AI centre. The presence of a sperm bank is more convenient in that it enables the whole donation of semen to be stored (sufficient for use on several occasions), and avoids the need for the donor to present fresh semen at the time the potential AID mother ovulates. The inconvenience of producing semen on demand has obvious unattractive implications. The donor may not be feeling particularly well or it may be otherwise inconvenient to supply the semen at a given time. The process of masturbation to order during a working day is not an activity that most men would consider satisfactory, and only the most dedicated, or irresponsible, donors are able to cope with such demands if they are frequently made. The donor is also asked to abstain from sexual activity for a period of time before the semen is collected and the inconvenience of this may be considerable. Over and above this the donor is faced with the difficulty of finding a suitable place to provide fresh semen during the day. This is not the clinical procedure many imagine but often requires the donor to masturbate into a container when hiding away from his colleagues, so the most obvious place is in a cubicle of the men's lavatory. The donation of semen is not as straightforward or as easy to arrange as it might appear.

The use of frozen semen has the added advantage of permitting a greater degree of impersonality than when fresh semen is used. The frozen semen is collected by a technician or the AI practitioner directly from a phial stored in a cylinder containing liquid nitrogen. Seen in this way the process is more detached and impersonal. Compare this with the elaborate procedures involved in the delivery of fresh semen from the donor to the AI practitioner. Sometimes more than one person is involved in its delivery. Leaving receptacles containing the semen on shelves, against doors and even behind geranium pots, to be picked up by the next person involved in the delivery system, is not unknown. The desire to keep the donor away from the AID mother and perhaps even from the AI practitioner leads to practices which can only be described as furtive.

The payment of donors may also be associated with the issues of availability and the need to depersonalise the process of collecting semen. But some argue that making a payment for semen merely exacerbates an already difficult situation both morally and practically. It is possible that a donor may hide important information which he believes will terminate the use of his semen if this might lead to the loss of his fee. This is a clear combination of the moral and practical issues involved in payment. If one is paid for a service of some kind, does the careful assessment of the reasons for providing the service remain as strong as when one gives the service freely? If, through the mechanism of payment, the donor is encouraged to put aside doubts he might otherwise have about donating semen, it could be said that payment has directly interfered with his assessment of the consequences of his act.

Whether receiving payment or not the donor occupies the position in the AID process which is probably the hardest to justify. To some observers, the willingness to provide semen in the way described automatically raises suspicion about the motives of the donor. Why does he do it? Does he really consider the outcome of his action? Does he ever have any regrets or doubts? Most of these questions are unanswerable at the present time mainly because it has not been possible to talk to more than a very few donors. The available information suggests that most donors have no thoughts about their action and they have no regrets whatsoever; 'it's the same as giving blood' is a common response. Yet of all the people involved, some claim that the donor is both morally and legally in the least defensible position (Dunstan, 1975).

Both the husband of the AID mother and the donor are 'fathers' in some sense but there are differences. The donor is a biological father and according to social custom has a clear responsibility for the children he has helped to create. There is no getting away from the fact that the genetic make-up of the resulting child created by the fusion of one of his sperm with an ovum of the child's mother owes as much to him as to her. In every other situation where a child's biological father is known, that father is expected and often required to fulfil certain obligations towards that child. The fact that sexual intercourse in the accepted sense of that term did not take place is irrelevant. A biological father can, of course, choose to allow his children to be adopted by someone else but this is usually done openly with the wider society taking special precautions to ensure that the interests of the child are properly represented. This is not the case with AID where knowledge of the procedure is usually confined to a very small group indeed. The moral responsibility of the donor in relation to the child cannot be simply removed by denying its importance and by using procedures which make his identification virtually impossible.

In the Norwegian study referred to in Chapter 2 one AID couple, when considering the donor, commented: 'To look upon a man as morally high-minded when going to breed children he does not especially want or for whom he has no responsibility seems to us somewhat absurd.' Løveset, the AI practitioner conducting this study, was not sympathetic to this view and added after the above comment: 'It is difficult to see why anybody should feel hurt by the use of his semen to help other people.' Løveset appears to miss the point the couple were making. The donor is *not* giving semen to help other people in the same way that many of us donate blood. Semen is being given for the purpose of *creating a new human being* whereas blood is given to assist those who are already in existence and who need help. The issues of personal and social responsibility surrounding the care of people who already exist are very different from those surrounding the planned creation of a new individual.

Legally the position is far from clear at the present time. Though it may appear to be an unlikely occurrence, it is possible that should the AID child, or indeed the AID mother, ascertain the identity of the donor, then the child has a right to maintenance by the donor in the same way that any other child has the right to support from its biological father. We believe that it is unlikely that the AI practitioner could be required to divulge the name of the donor where this is known, but it is interesting to notice that members of the legal profession acting as advisers to their medical colleagues have suggested that medical practitioners providing AID should protect themselves by using consent forms for both the AID couple and the donor. A form has been designed for *donor consent* in addition to forms signifying consent by the AID couple.

Listing the practical, personal, legal and moral issues facing the AI donor serves to demonstrate the ambiguity of his position. He regularly provides semen in a way which most would consider to be inconvenient, embarrassing and perhaps even sordid. He does this because he is requested to do so by a person whom he respects or because he is receiving a fee. There is no apparent underlying personal need as in the case of the childless couple; indeed the criteria for donor selection indicate that a potential donor who possessed an obvious and stated desire to sire unknown children for psychological reasons of his own would be refused the opportunity. Perhaps this is why those inquiring into AID have made such statements as:

> We feel that the role of donor is of such a kind that it is liable to appeal to the abnormal and unbalanced . . . Whether the lack of responsibility which, in our view, is likely to characterise the process of donation of semen, however well balanced the donor may other-wise be, is liable to be passed on to the child must, however, be open to doubt.
>
> (Feversham Committee, 1960)

The belief that such unacceptable traits may not be inherited is used to reduce the unease concerning this particular issue, but a feeling of uncertainty about it nevertheless remains.

THE DONOR AND THE AID COUPLE

It is not always the case that the AID couple are unaware of the identity of the donor but this is usually so. Sometimes a request for a specific donor such as a cousin or a brother of the husband has been made but these appear to be very rare. Cases of deliberate deception by the husband as to the identity of the donor have occurred and have been reported (see Chapter 2) but these are remembered because they are exceptions to the general rule. Where a couple insist on a particular type of donor in an attempt to ensure that the AID child will possess certain physical or mental characteristics, this is sometimes taken as a contraindication of the suitability of the couple for AID (Kerr and Rogers, 1975). Again we see the AID practitioner acting as the filter in the relationship between the AID couple and the donor.

One commentator casts an interesting light on the relationship between the AID couple and the donor as controlled by the AI practitioner. He indicates that the responsibilities do not flow in a single direction.

As the physician is asking the donor not only to give his seed but also to relinquish all ethical and parental responsibilities which he may feel for the child his seed produces, the doctor should be able to assure the donor that the couple receiving AID will be able to care for the child produced.

(Richards, 1971)

This is a fine sentiment but it raises the question of how this assurance is to be given and assumes that the donor has such an interest. Our own information suggests that the whole AID process is based on an unstated assumption of trust in the AI practitioner.

Couples do have an interest in the physical characteristics and mental attributes of the donor *before* AID is begun, but this interest is apparently suppressed once the AID process has started. If success is obtained and a pregnancy is achieved, the role of the donor is sometimes played down or occasionally denied by the couple. This desire to forget the donor or make no reference to him once the AID process has begun is a common phenomenon. In one large AID practice the AI practitioner reports that on only one occasion (in forty years) has a mother sent a present for the donor on the birth of her child (although it is a common occurrence for mothers to send flowers to the AI practitioner). Clearly most AID mothers prefer to put the thought of the donor out of their heads.

The donor is sometimes mentioned when couples are considering a second AID child; many ask for the same donor. This request may simply be a response to the perceived success with the first AID child but it is possible that it has much deeper significance than this. One couple, after having two children by AID, wrote seeking confirmation that the two children were 'full blood brothers'. This suggests that the desire to maintain the family unit as a cohesive one with the minimum of different extra-familial blood ties is important to some people.

Apart from this interest in the donor when seeking a second AID child, it was noted that there is some interest in him before AID begins. Assurances concerning the ethnic origins of the donor are often requested. There are Jewish couples who request a Jewish donor and non-Jewish couples who request a non-Jewish donor. There are some husbands who demand an Englishman, or Scotsman, or Welshman, and there are those who list donor types who would not be acceptable. Even the request for a patriotic donor is not unknown. This desire for a donor with certain characteristics highlights the difficulty facing those in minority racial groups when attempting to obtain AID in this country; a difficulty which is due to the greater scarcity of available males and the presence of cultural and religious taboos which prevent their involvement.

4

The AID Child

When discussing the relationships between those involved in the AID process, the child needs to be put in a special category. There is a significant difference between taking part in the *creation* of the child by means of artificial insemination and being the *result* of that process. In our view much of the current debate about AID is based on a false premiss relating directly to the AID child. The false premiss is the often-stated belief that it is the child who is of primary concern when AID is being undertaken.

The AID child is undoubtedly a planned child. Of all children, this is one feature that marks him out. Thus conception has followed careful planning which has entailed uncomfortable and possibly embarrassing procedures, often after years of longing for a child. This is no child of passion. Some potential AID parents abandon the attempt, finding the procedure too clinical, whilst others continue trying each month, sometimes year after year, in the hope that a child may be conceived. In many years of research into fertility-regulating behaviour we have never before been made so aware of the depth of longing and need by individuals and couples as found among those who desire a child and who, for one reason or another, are denied the opportunity of having one.

The AID child is almost always both a planned *and* a

wanted child. Many letters confirming this have been received from satisfied parents:

> our baby has turned our house into a home full of happiness. I hope you will continue to make other couples as happy and proud as my husband and myself . . .

And again,

> you can imagine how happy [we] feel after waiting for this to happen for such a long time . . . I can hardly believe it has really happened to me.

The wanting and planning of these children are obvious. There are very many such satisfied couples. This appreciation is not just confined to having a *baby*. Those who have grown-up children are equally strong in their feelings that they 'did the right thing'. One mother who wrote after her AID children were adults and had left home to set up homes of their own makes this clear:

> There is nothing that we would change in any way – they have given us such a happy family life . . . we think they have developed into well-balanced adults.

Some observers have suggested that because of the willingness of AID parents, and especially mothers, to go to such lengths to become parents, the resulting child may be overindulged or one or both parents will become overpossessive of the child. It is true that reference to the physical similarities, traits, mannerisms and even attitudes which link the child to the husband are often stressed. One researcher has suggested that claims for such similarities are much more frequent in the AID family than in other families but this is perhaps indicative of the strong psychological need to appear as a 'normal' family rather than the result of undue posses-siveness. The evidence made available to us indicates that by far the majority of AID families are stable and emotionally secure.

It has been said that the AID child is at an advantage when compared to other children in that his origins are not the result of some chance meeting or some moment of passion. By a process of careful selection the AID child is getting a calculated inheritance which suggests that the child will be as good as, if not better than, normally conceived children. In addition the family environment in which the child is to be reared has been assessed and also considered to be satisfactory. Not all children have the benefit of the combination of this favourable heredity and environmental background so it can be seen that when a child is planned in this way the claim that the child will be 'superior' is based on a eugenic belief that selective breeding will somehow enrich the human race.

When selective breeding takes place, passing on of high-quality genetic material is emphasised, but in AID there is an added dimension in that not only are biological parents being selected but 'social' parents with whom the child will grow up are also selected. The careful combining of bio-logical and environmental factors ('nature' and 'nurture') is undertaken in such a way that we may ask: cannot only good come of it? Could a child ask for a better start in life than this?

The issues of AID parent and donor selection have already been raised in previous chapters and the determination of what constitutes a 'good' biological or environmental back-ground has been shown to be more idiosyncratic and un-certain than many would suppose. How are the 'better chances' and the 'superiority' of the AID child to be assessed? And more important, for whose benefit is the selection of AID parents (both biological and social), and the process as a whole, being undertaken? Some researchers (e.g. Iizuka *et al.*, 1968) have claimed that the AID child demonstrates superior physical and mental qualities yet nothing is said of emotional stability, contentedness and sense of fulfilment on the part of the child. Doubtless many AID parents would argue that their own child possesses these attributes but this is usually in an environment where the child is kept in ignorance of his true origins. If eugenic arguments are being put forward it could be claimed that it is society as a whole that will benefit from AID in that 'good stock' is being encouraged. The only place where such arguments are raised appears to be in articles and papers describing the work of AI practitioners where the positive outcomes of AID are listed in order, perhaps, to justify AID at the social as well as the personal level. It is at the personal level that AID is important to childless couples who come to the AI practitioner in expectation of having their need satisfied. At this level it is the AID parents, the mother and her husband, who are being helped. AID is being used to benefit them in a way that no other procedure or treatment can. The child cannot be a beneficiary at this stage because at the time AID is being considered the child does not exist! The argument that the child is going to be given a 'good start' through the process of parental selection, and that this is therefore of direct benefit to the child, is a specious one.

There is nothing novel in this. The AID child is no different from any other child in that he has no choice as to who his parents will be. In most societies, including our own, inadequate parentage is a well-known phenomenon. The AID child may have an advantage in that the risk of being presented with inadequate parents is likely to be less than for other children. However, it is not the parent/child relationship which is at issue here but the procedures surrounding that relationship. The most regularly stated claim by those who have studied AID, whether these be government committees, medical working parties, religious commissions, individual AI practitioners, or other observers, is that before embarking on the AID process the outcome for the child should be the primary consideration. It is apparent that our thinking about this issue is confused. Public statements are being made about the care of a non-existent child in order to allay fears about the procedure which will lead to the creation of this, as yet, non-existent child. How can we possibly justify in such circumstances the statement that the child is benefiting from AID?

If AID is being resorted to for the sake of the mother or her husband, then let us say so and not pretend that the concern for the parents comes second to that for the child. This is an important point for if we really believe that it is the child who is our primary concern, then the whole issue of keeping that child in ignorance of his or her true origins and of setting up procedures to ensure that such ignorance is maintained needs to be examined very carefully. Moreover, the retention of a legal situation which labels the child as illegitimate and which encourages those involved to act in an illegal way requires reassessment. If we really mean to consider AID from the child's point of view then a totally different perspective on AID emerges: a perspective which is likely to call into question many of the established procedures and accepted ways of thinking about AID.

Who, then, speaks for the child in this situation? The adopted child has the benefit of a legal framework which prescribes certain processes and designates certain officials to assist in the adoption in the child's interest. The AID child however has no such benefit and whilst decisions in many cases may be the result of care, sometimes they can be idiosyncratic. Thus the AID child differs from the adopted child, the illegitimate child and the child born into a normal family setting. Here is the basic issue which permeates all discussion of AID – a child is being created! It is not a question of coping, in the kindest possible way, with a child who already exists, and who needs support, sustenance, warmth and love, but one who is not yet in being. Such a child is by no means an 'accident' or at the time of conception unwanted. The child is planned very carefully and such planning involves active participation by three people and usually the support of a fourth.

If our prime concern should be for the child, it might be thought there would be a follow-up of the AID family but usually interest ceases with the achievement of conception. Many AI practitioners do not even inquire about the outcome of the pregnancy, preferring to remove themselves from the scene as soon as a conception using donated semen has taken place. Others continue to have an interest but such a follow-up is not usually undertaken in a systematic way. Indeed, it is difficult to obtain unbiased information from such observations which would enable us to reach some valid conclusion about the effect of AID on the developing child.

This raises the issue of what constitutes success? If policy decisions are to be made concerning the practice of AID some knowledge of the results of the practice are necessary. Yet at the present time there is very little information about the effect AID has on the resulting family and the child. The Archbishop of Canterbury's commission reporting as long ago as 1948 said:

My Commission observed, very truly, that as yet there is little evidence available upon which to judge the sociological and psychological effects of AID. There are too few observed cases and too few cases observed for a sufficient length of time.

And the Feversham Committee, reporting in 1960:

there is no doubt that all discussion of the practice is at present greatly handicapped by lack of information about what has subsequently happened to the families of those women who have received AID . . .

80

The medical profession in the form of the Peel Committee reported in 1973:

> The Panel has had evidence from several sources urging that, for psychological reasons, there should be no follow-up of children born to AID. It understands but does not entirely agree with these views. Information must be obtained on the genetic effects especially where frozen semen has been used and it is important to learn the effects, in human terms, on the development of personal relationships in families resulting from the use of AID.

This agreement on the part of government officials and by those representing the clerical and medical professions is worth noting. Whilst not denying the difficulties inherent in such a study, we would support the view that this information should be acquired. The co-ordination of AI practitioners' work has been attempted by the Royal College of Obstetricians and Gynaecologists but its concern has been more to do with the task of setting up an AID service rather than with the social and psychological results of the service. Some centres, and individuals, have undertaken small-scale studies but these have been generally of limited scope. The most imaginative to date is a study in one centre where successful AID parents are being asked to forward colour photographs of the child at 1, 3 and 7 years of age. Follow-up social reports are also planned. Presumably the photographs are to be compared with those of the husband and/or the donor but this is not explicitly stated. In any event, whilst physical resemblance (or rather the lack of physical resemblance) may appear to be of particular interest to those seeking donors, in a rapidly changing donor population it is difficult to see how such photographic follow-up is to be used. The added difficulty in maintaining confidentiality with the AID parents, anonymity of the donor and secrecy in relation to the child that a photographic record introduces we presume must also have been considered.

How long should one wait before pronouncing whether AID has, or has not, been a success in any given instance, and from whom should such information be collected? Horne, an American AI practitioner writing in 1975, argued that success or failure of the AID process should not be measured by the pregnancy rate alone, nor even the experience of the child's early life but

> also by the long range sociologic and psychologic effect on both the infertile couple and the child, as revealed a generation later. Until now, there appears to have been no such long range study reported in the scientific literature. Until 25 years have passed and the treated couples and at least some of their artificially induced offspring have been questioned, the rightness or wrongness of AID will not become clear.

We know what he means, but 'a generation later'? How is such a study to be mounted and how will the AID children be identified and questioned?

KEEPING THE AID SECRET FROM THE CHILD

Any study which purports to assess the impact of AID on the child must deal with the problems of identifying a reasonable number of such children who are aware of their AID status. This may prove very difficult to achieve for almost all AID children, as far as we are able to tell, are unaware of their origins. Most AID parents keep the secret of AID from their child or children and apparently have no intention of ever revealing it. We have already seen in Chapter 2 that occasionally the fact of AID is revealed to the child as a result of marital instability of some kind. The child in such circumstances is made aware of AID either indirectly, for example, during divorce proceedings, or more directly when the child is used by one partner in the marriage to hurt the other. It is worth stressing that whilst such cases are rare nevertheless they do occasionally occur. Even more rare is the situation where the AID parents are known to have voluntarily informed the child of his or her origins.

Comparison with adoption procedures is again brought to mind here. In the case of adoption, adoptive parents are strongly advised to inform the child of his of her adopted status and a legal framework is available which gives the child certain rights about ascertaining his or her biological parentage at the age of 18 years. This is not so in relation to AID, and AID parents are often counselled by AI practitioners not to divulge such information to the child. In one obvious respect, the AID child is more a 'natural' child of the family than the adopted child yet parents are encouraged to deny information to the AID child and encouraged to provide it to the adopted child. There appears to be a genuine fear among AI practitioners that to reveal the truth to the AID child will create adverse social and psychological reactions for both the family as a whole and for the child concerned. This may, in part, explain why follow-up of AID couples and children has not been generally undertaken. However, the deception necessary to keep the child in ignorance of his true origins is now being questioned by some AI practitioners.

It is becoming recognised that the social and psychological problems created by keeping the secret from the child (and by implication, other members of the family) may be greater than those that result from telling the child. It should be remembered that similar views were expressed before legislation was passed in relation to the adoption of children. On the one hand there are the problems implicit in deception, problems which might increase rather than decrease with time as the child grows up, and on the other hand there are the rights of the child to have information about his origins where these are known. Merely following a procedure which makes certain that the child's origins remain obscure does not resolve this issue if the procedure has been planned with the mother's and her husband's agreement.

Deceiving the child is claimed by some to be the kindest and most loving thing to do for the child because by this means the child is being protected from possible discrimination, and mental stress. To explain the fact of AID to a young child, it is argued, would be very difficult and if it is left until the child is an adult it is suggested that the outcome could be very damaging, as evidence from adoption studies indicates. It is for such reasons that some AI practitioners advise parents not to tell the child, and to forget about AID once the child is conceived. Others, perhaps a little less certain, believe that the decision whether or not to tell the child should be left to the AID couple, offering no opinion one way or the other themselves. One leaflet for would-be AID parents puts this very clearly:

> Unless you decide to tell the child there is no reason for him (or her) ever to know that he (or she) was conceived by AID. Whether or not you do so is entirely up to you.
>
> (RCOG, 1979b)

The role of the AI practitioner is important here for many couples appear to accept almost without question the advice to forget all about it. The high professional status of the AI practitioner and the deep desire of the couples to appear normal constitute a powerful combination encouraging wishful thinking and self-deception. Nevertheless, it is sometimes not at all easy to keep such a secret from the child.

Communication is not only dependent on the spoken word; sometimes there exists an unspoken awareness that a particular topic should be avoided. Even young children can sense this without there ever being direct mention of it. This is particularly so in the family, which is an organisation where each person has the opportunity to get to know the feelings and thoughts of other members who are regularly in close proximity. We adjust to these feelings almost unconsciously but there are occasions when they can be very intrusive. It would not be hard for most of us to find examples of this in our own families.

There are two points here that are relevant to the AID family: first, the secret may not be as secure as the family would like to believe and, secondly, security may become more difficult as the child grows up and becomes more discerning. We have already noted how some mothers (a very small number, admittedly) are reported as refusing drugs at the time of the AID child's birth for fear of unwittingly divulging the secret of the child's conception to those in attendance. Children, too, are sometimes aware that there is a deep family secret without knowing the precise nature of the secret. Sometimes the fantasy surrounding the secret takes very strange forms such as those reported by Gerstel who, when treating five AID families for psychological disturbance, discovered that some of the children believed they were the result of virgin births. Without talking to the children directly an assessment of how they think about themselves and about others in the family can only remain conjecture at the present time. All the information relating to the child given above has been obtained from others – usually the AID parents who are speaking on behalf of the child.

THE AID CHILD

The final section of this chapter is devoted to a selection from three letters about AID; the first is written by an adopted child and the other two by AID children. Two have been taken from letters sent to a national newspaper and the other was sent directly to one of the authors. As these letters are being read it is worth reconsidering the two related issues concerning the benefits of AID and justification for keeping secret the origins of the AID child. How should the responsibility for bringing an AID child into the world be shared between the parents, the AI practitioner, the donor and society at large? Who should be responsible for deciding which households should receive an AID child, bearing in mind the current availability of AID to married couples, homosexual couples and single women? Here is a *Guardian* reader's reply to a couple contemplating AID:

Dear Mr and Mrs Ex,
You are considering whether to go ahead with AID. *Please don't.* You find important the fact that the child would be the flesh and blood of one of you – but what about the other? I hope that the child would *not* be considered by the 'unnatural' father as his 'very own'. A child is not something to acquire – it is not property.

I write as a happily married 40 year old with two teenage boys. What can I know of the longing that you have for a baby in your arms? What I do know, however, is the sadness and emotion of looking at my children and worrying why they do this; why they react in this way; how do I guide them when one side of their inheritance is an unknown quantity.

Why am I like I am – who am I? I discovered my natural mother two years ago as a result of the new Adopted Children's Act – she was related to my known family but my father remains 'anonymous' although I search for his likeness in crowds, outside the Salvation Army hostel, on television, everywhere. So that is my identity crisis and it's very hard to bear. I wish my father would pop up from 'nowhere'.

I cannot forget that I was brought up living a lie – I was never told I was adopted but the secret did come out and, I feel, spoilt two lives in the attempts to keep it. I am horrified to read that it is thought that the child gains nothing from the truth in this instance. We must never let honesty become an irrelevant policy . . . It is a wise child who knows its own father but please, there are enough of us who don't know who we are already.

(*Guardian*, 5 July 1979)

Another reader wrote:

. . . My father (or nearest available equivalent as I was actually born by AID) left when I was three years old, leaving me to be brought up by my mother on her own. It was a horribly lonely childhood. In my case, it maybe wasn't her fault, but the experience left me with a lot of ambivalent feelings towards her and towards women in general. I resented being so emotionally dependent on mother; at the same time I needed her badly just because she was the only parent, and cried one hell of a lot when she left me in the charge of other women to go out to work.

If 'avoiding the patriarchal family structure' means that women are going to deliberately have babies on their own, calling in a floating population of male and female baby-minders, as they please, this is just not good enough. The legal norm should be two close parents at least, with every parent having equal control. If that means that women have less power than they otherwise would – well, there are other things that matter besides female power . . .

(*Guardian*, 24 May 1979)

In the covering letter attached to the following statement, the writer observed: 'enough has been written about the legality of birth certificates and far too little about feelings'. This 24-year-old AID child asked that her experience should be shared with others:

. . . My mother conceived me by AID. My 'father' had, according to my mother, never shown any interest in sex or, indeed, physical contact of any kind . . . All this was alluded to me by the time I was four: in addition she said that as he was unable to 'put his seed into her, a doctor had put it there with a test tube', or words to that effect. I remember the discussion quite clearly for I wished to know exactly what a test tube looked like . . .

I knew that somehow my sister did not belong to 'us' – mum never described a pregnancy, birth, or breast-feeding with regard to my sister. By careful cross-questioning I extracted the information that my sister was adopted – she was told a year later. But never once did it enter my head that he whom we called my dad was not my real father. Grandmother [maternal] would note my resemblance to him whenever I lost my temper, neighbours would look me in the eyes, examine me minutely and remark how much I took after my father . . .

Mum decided that the truth must be revealed for I was developing, would soon be a woman. She was too embarrassed, I suppose, to tell me herself and she asked her lover of five years to explain the facts of my life to me . . . He sat me on his lap while mum stood anxiously behind. He asked if I knew about cows being 'injected' with test tubes of sperm – I said that of course I did, never being one to admit ignorance. There was obviously something more to all this but I still did not predict what was to come next. 'That's the way your mum fell for you.' There must have been more questions from me, answers from him but essentially I felt like escaping, carrying this great, shattering boulder of information away with me.

I had a picture of grunting farm animals, test tubes, sperm and me. God the father had deserted me, I was the child of the devil: a pubescent melodrama that I acted out in hate and revenge.

In the months that followed I attempted to flesh out my biological father. My mother supplied the only information that she had. To make sure that his sperm was 'all right' every donor had to have three children. Somewhere I had more family. He had to be of good moral character, so I should be reassured that there was nothing of the criminal in my blood. He was probably a policeman, possibly a doctor . . .

Never did I worry about being a bastard. No, what upset my whole sense of being was that nobody knew my 'real' father: as though half of me did not, does not exist.

But my mother clearly felt a sense of shame for I was sworn to secrecy. Therefore I told everybody the circumstances of my conception at the earliest opportunity. I sought out my most garrulous cousin and told her 'everything', in return for her juicy family secrets. She spread the news throughout my mother's family. To this day maternal aunts, who showed me affection in my early years, dislike and ignore me. Doubtless my personality has contributed greatly to this state of affairs but I do wonder . . . My grandmother always finds occasion to speak darkly about 'blood' in my company, blood and its mysterious capacity to 'carry' talents and traits. She always knew just how my mother had conceived me for she had paid the necessary fee for my conception.

My father died of Huntingdon's Chorea four years ago. Mother's family commiserated warmly with my sister and all but ignored me. They knew logically I was no carrier of the dreadful disease but my 'father's' family have never been told. They avoided my eyes, pretended I did not exist. Thank God that an anonymous donor, with good blood, is my father and not a carrier of Huntingdon's Chorea.

That would be the end of the 'information' I have to offer but for one queer twist of fate . . . I married early and in the manner of the majority of adolescent girls who have no career, no alternative model, I longed for a baby. None came. After all the long drawn out tests we were told, or rather I was told, 'Your husband has no spermatozoa – he is sterile'. I was eighteen and the question of AID came to my mind in a new light. In discussions with my mother it came out that she had worried about what she was carrying when pregnant, had looked at me and wondered about my origins, my father, from whom I had inherited all undesirable traits . . .

Subsequently I . . . came to understand my mother's decision to have a baby by AID. She was no thoughtless ogre but a woman who craved her own child. But me, how can I make such a decision? My child would lack two generations of fathers. I could not hide the circumstances of my own conception for it might well find out about my 'father's' inherited illness and be full of fear. Friends and relatives all know that my husband is sterile (he has had a biopsy to confirm that his condition is irreversible). Children sense the unsaid – it would have to be told and told young. My husband and I have been unable to resolve the dilemma. Instead I went to Teacher Training College and now teach nursery children thus detracting from my desire for children, not that this helps my husband in any way.

One thing I do know – the initials AID come to haunt me every day of my life.

5

The AID Family

We have so far looked at the relationships between five people: the couple, the AID child, the AI practitioner and the donor. In so doing we have touched on the problems of confidentiality existing between the couple and the AI practitioner, the anonymity of the donor and the secrecy surrounding the AID child. In this chapter we shall explore these problems further but with emphasis on the AID family as a unit. The relationship of the AID family to wider kinsfolk, friends, neighbours and even society at large is important in any understanding of the social affects of AID.

When discussing the AID family it is of immediate concern to consider the means by which the fact of AID is dealt with. We have already seen that the normal procedure is to keep AID secret. This secrecy may be viewed at three levels: first, there is the parents' concern to keep the child ignorant of his AID origins; secondly, there is the concealment of the nature of the paternity from the wider kin of which the family is a part; and thirdly, there is the issue of secrecy surrounding the whole practice of AID in our society at the present time. Here we shall examine the AID secret with regard to near relatives, more distant relatives, friends and neighbours.

Essentially, the problem facing the AID family is one of paternity. A child has been born to the wife through donated semen. The husband and wife, in confidence, consented to artificial insemination and the anonymous donor willingly provided semen. So how are we to regard the relationship between the husband and the donor? In the English language surprisingly we are short of words to make a distinction; surprisingly, for in many other areas of discourse we have a rich vocabulary. In Latin, however, there are two words and we should get used to them. The *genitor* is the biological connection, the male who provided the sperm which fertilised the ovum in the female. In this case the donor is the genitor. The *pater* is the father, that is to say, the male who is legally responsible for the child's welfare, the person to whom the child owes filial obedience and who presides usually as head of the household. In the normal family the pater and genitor are one and the same person. In some cases, however, they are not the same. Thus a husband may be a step-father to his wife's children because they were the offspring of a previous marriage, or he may be the adopting father of either his wife's or more often another woman's child who has legally been given to him and his wife for adoption and whose status has been officially recorded in the adoption register. As pointed out in Chapter 1 in the family created by AID the pater usually pretends to be the genitor but in fact he is not, whereas in the case of step-, foster or adopted chidren no pretence is made in law and in most instances not in the family and the community. We have, therefore, to ask precisely: 'What is the content of paternity?' If we can answer this question we shall perhaps be able to shed light on the nature of the secrecy which appears so essential to AID and which permeates any consideration of it.

We may begin by saying that because we only have the one word *father* in our language most people associate together the roles of both *genitor* and *pater*, and for general purposes this confusion is without difficulty or disadvantage. If we analyse the concept of fatherhood we find it to be a 'role-complex', which is to say that of fathers we expect several things. We normally expect them to be the genitor and where not we expect this to be made explicit, but we also expect other things and in the family these are important expectations. Thus the father is a male and his masculinity is a model for a boy to note and copy, or at least learn to approximate to more and more as he grows up. He is also a model for a girl to know what masculinity is in contrast to her femininity for which model she takes her mother. The father is, as we have indicated, the head of the household, symbolised very often by his sitting at the 'head' of the table, taking the lead in decision-making, and usually acting as final court of appeal in family quarrels and disputes. But there is much more than this, for father has also a socio-legal role to play. He has legal rights and obligations with regard to the child's welfare. He provides through his work the wherewithal by which the family lives and he represents the family in the community. He may even have a quasi-priestly and pastoral role to play. In ancient Greece the father *was* a priest, for the ancient religion of the hearth entailed his performing ceremonies, pouring libations to the ancestors and saying the words of worship and supplication. Indeed, originally in the Ancient World adoption was an institution designed to provide a family which was without a son with one who would succeed to the familial priestly office on the father's death. If this seems far removed from the present day let it nevertheless be said that fathers are often expected to give counsel, advice and comfort to members of the family in distress; to advise in a matter of conscience or of concern for others, to help a family member in a dilemma or personal difficulty; in short, there is a pastoral role.

How does all this affect the AID family? Let us approach the task indirectly. Consider the case of a woman with children whose husband has left her. Another adult male comes to live with her and her children. Will he be called 'father'? Almost certainly he will not, for the children will know he is not the father and so will neighbours and friends. However, he may well fulfil some paternal roles. He may be a model of masculinity, provide an income and act as head of the house, and even fulfil a pastoral role. But he will not fulfil the socio-legal role because he is not married to the woman. Two important ingredients in the paternal role are missing; he is neither the genitor nor the legally responsible pater.

The husband of the AID mother may well fulfil all roles but one. He cannot without deception play the role of genitor, for that has been played by the donor. The donor, however, has not been allowed to accept any paternal role other than this, nor would he generally wish to do so. There are very good reasons why the donor would not wish to be known to the AID child he has helped to create. There are legal responsibilities under current English law which donors would incur. Paternity could be claimed, their estates could be distributed on their death to the offspring they have sired.

It is this deception connected with paternity which is the source of all secrecy surrounding the practice of AID. It could be said that keeping the child in ignorance of its genetic origin, ensuring the donor remains anonymous, undertaking the AID process in a clandestine atmosphere and even keeping the fact of AID from friends, neighbours and relatives stems from this fundamental issue of paternity. There should be no doubt about the desire for secrecy. Both husbands and wives write to AI practitioners urging them to destroy records, and not to engage in correspondence with them.

The secret is not restricted to the husband alone. It is shared with at least two people: the wife and the AI practitioner. The wife is a willing party to the secret because she wants a child, possibly she wants a child because her husband wants one, and there is some evidence that the husband often takes the initiative in this matter. Sometimes the wife is inseminated by a mixture of semen from both husband and donor. Again, advice is often given to a couple to have sexual intercourse as soon after and preferably on the same day that AID is taking place. An advice leaflet distributed by the Royal College of Obstetricians and Gynaecologists says:

> babies born within a marriage are presumed to be legitimate and provided you do not abstain from intercourse during the period in which AID was carried out there can be no certainty that any child conceived is not your husband's.
>
> (RCOG, 1979b)

This mixing of semen and the recommendation to have sexual intercourse the same day that AID takes place is sometimes claimed as being beneficial to the husband for psychological reasons. The husband may receive some psychological comfort by being directly involved physiologically or behaviourally in the creation of the child, but it is also worth noting that the RCOG advice also makes it extremely difficult to prove in law that the husband was not the *genitor* of the child. This advice reveals some difficulty for the husband who is deliberately refraining from being the genitor because of rhesus incompatibility or because he carries known harmful genetic factors. In such cases the husband and wife have undertaken AID not because the husband is sterile but because of the dangers to the potential child if his own sperm is used. The presumption in such cases is that the husband is not the genitor and the attempt to confuse the legal situation is therefore weakened. Even if the psychological or legal reasons for such advice are honestly held, it remains difficult to avoid the charge that deception of some sort is being encouraged.

The advantages of having a highly qualified professional person to act as an intermediary between the couple seeking AID and the donor were discussed in Chapter 2. The AI practitioner who fulfils this role provides a feeling of confidence that the secret of AID will be kept. Yet one has to ask just how well kept the couple's secret is. To be sure it will be easier to keep it if the AI practitioner is working in a large city rather than in a small town or a village. It will be easier if the patients travel some distance for AID, and if the anonymous donors are not permanently resident in the area. We have seen that medical students most often act as donors; they are held to be intelligent and healthy, they are also mobile and they are being trained for a profession which has a high regard for confidentiality. However, information of a confidential kind can nevertheless get about. A conference paper by G. L. Foss, mentioned in an RCOG study report in 1976, referred to the lack of confidentiality of medical records, in particular those stored in health centres. On several occasions AID mothers had complained that they had been embarrassed by reference to their babies being conceived by a donor instead of their husband. The comment was made, 'when the husband visits one can only imagine how he feels about this flagrant lack of confidentiality'. It is difficult to see how, as public health practice takes over from private practice, confidentiality can be maintained at a high level, for the bureaucratic machinery and the impersonality of the relationships which such bureaucracy engenders militate against it.

The purpose of examining yet again the relationships between the AID couple, the donor and the AI practitioner is to demonstrate that confidentiality, anonymity and secrecy in relation to AID cannot be maintained without serious deception. This deception is for the sole purpose of keeping the fact of AID from the community in which the AID family resides. This community includes friends, neighbours and others in addition to those who are closely related to the AID family. How are we to describe the family? Quite clearly it consists of something more than the mother, AID child and her husband; we shall leave out of consideration one-parent families for the present. There may be siblings – children of the mother by a previous husband or children fathered by the husband prior to his having had an irreversible vasectomy. But in addition both the husband and the wife may have siblings and also parents and parents' siblings; these wider kinsfolk are also in some sense part of the family. Of course, the manner in which they are regarded as family may vary greatly. Sometimes when we speak of family we mean the immediate two-generation group of parents and immature children, but often we think of family as including a wider range of kinsfolk. We do of course make a distinction between those in a given household and those who are outside it, and to be sure in our modern industrial and urbanised society the small two-generation family in a single household is usual. However, many households include one or more grandparents, usually elderly and retired. Family structure differs from town to country where relatives may be living in close proximity even if not in the same household. Urban dwellers tend to be more geographically mobile, and kinsfolk may be scattered over a wide area. Moreover, in many middle-class families geographical mobility is a function of occupational career patterns.

Thus the problems facing the AID family may be more or less intense according to how many kinsfolk they have, and how proximately they are situated to the AID family household. Yet there is a further social factor to be considered. This relates to people's customary expectations. Social norms are not uniform and what may be a normal expectation in one case may be different in another. Thus in traditional British working-class families there is often a close relationship between mother and daughter which continues after the daughter's marriage. Some observers (e.g. Kerr, 1958; Young and Willmott, 1962; Klein, 1965) recount how some married daughters regularly went home to 'Mum' and slept there. The mother also acted as baby-sitter and she and her daughter would often go shopping together.

Middle-class family patterns vary but some display a highly individualistic outlook; the parents leaving the married offspring alone, deliberately not interfering unless invited to do so. It is here that geographical distance may help to provide that independence from kinsfolk that some seek and others endure.

These differences in situation affect relationships within all families but they may have deeper significance for the AID family. Clearly, close proximity makes keeping secrets and maintaining confidentiality more difficult than distance; but equally there may be more or less inclination on the part of the parents of married offspring to be involved in or to be cognisant of the intimacies of family life. Geographical mobility may also make it easier to maintain confidentiality in relation to neighbours and friends. The mobile couple may establish friendly and neighbourly relationships with people in their community after the acquisition of an AID child with less fear of the child's status becoming known. This may be harder to achieve if the AID couple continue to live in the place where they themselves grew up and where they married.

A consideration of relationships between kinsfolk reveals immediately a variation of beliefs and practices, but there are some regularities; indeed, in most societies some of these are well defined. For example, in societies of a traditional kind the grandparents or a mother's brother may have clear rights and obligations with respect to their grandchildren or their nephews and nieces. Whilst such rigid and formal practices relating to the rights and obligations of grandparents and uncles are uncommon in modern society there is a host of informal rights and obligations affecting their relationships within the family. Within the two-generation family of parents and immature children the formal rights and obligations are usually upheld in law; the right to expect reasonable obedience from the child and the obligation to provide for his or her welfare are examples. When, however, we consider wider kin, rights and obligations are still present but they now tend to be informal. Whether formal or informal, such rights and obligations with the expectations which underlie them are very important. Grandparents do have a role to play even though they have no formal responsibility for the child's welfare, and the parent's siblings, both the husband's and the wife's, are cognisant of a special relationship with the child by virtue of their close kinship by blood or by marriage. The child will also grow up in the knowledge that some relationships are different from others and that closeness of kinship is of importance in governing both attitudes and behaviour towards other.

It is from these perceived 'rights' and 'obligations' of a formal or informal kind that people come to have expectations; expectations which are widely held in common. There may well be variations from one social class to another, they may differ from town to country, and there may be differences between the wife's kinsfolk and the husband's kinsfolk but nevertheless these expectations are generally shared.

Such expectations may obtain even when, in law, there are no formal rights. In our society the grandparents on both sides will usually feel they have a 'right' to have access to their grandchildren and their own children are 'obliged' to permit this access; in law of course they have no such rights, but despite this the expectations they hold will be strongly held. Such expectations in normal circumstances are upheld by public opinion, or as the sociologist says, the culture 'enjoins' certain kinds of behaviour. It will be appreciated that these expectations extend to other kinsfolk in addition to the grandparents. If a nephew appears on the doorstep of his uncle's house unkempt and impoverished, say, during a hiking holiday, and makes it known he could do with a small loan and a bed for the night, then the uncle is likely to acquiesce, where a non-kinsman might well give the young fellow short shrift. This reflects the nephew's expectations regarding his uncle's willingness to co-operate. The uncle plays his part by fulfilling the role that he feels is expected of him.

Just as we examined the 'father' or paternal role and attempted to disentangle some of the ingredients of that role-complex, so we may examine the roles of the grand-parent, the uncle, the aunt, the nephew or niece, the son or daughter, and so on. The grandparental role is particularly prominent owing to the task of 'keeping the family together' which usually devolves on them. It is held to be beneficial for the family to keep in contact, to remind adult offspring of the desirability of offering help to, and receiving help from, various members of the family, symbolised by Christmas gifts and the recognition of birthdays and other anniversaries. Grandparents tend also to 'preside' over families even when geographically separated. Should the parents of a child die then an uncle or an aunt or other close relative would probably care for the orphaned child. A child may even expect to inherit property from a grandparent or from an uncle or aunt without issue.

What links all these activities are the 'expectations' which underlie them. Expectations can be immediately apparent, realised only under special circumstances or left dormant until long after a new member of the family is born. As the child grows so the expectations of kinfolk and others multiply. These expectations are based on trust and on the usually unstated belief that one's kinsfolk are related in the same way they – and other kinsfolk – say they are. But what if such relationships are based on a deception; a deception shared by some members of the family kin but not others? The key factor in the AID process is the maintenance of secrecy of the child's genetic origins. In most cases it is not only the child who is being kept in ignorance of these origins.

As the AID child grows up it is probable that close relatives of the AID couple begin individually to establish personal relationships with the child. It is as the child gets older that the relationships with wider kin assume some significance, rather than at birth or in the period immediately following. All the time these relationships are being developed there is a state of trust between the AID couple and their kinsfolk, confidence in the tacit understanding, unquestioned and unquestionable, that the uncle of the child is really the uncle and the child his nephew or niece, that the grandfather and grandmother are the grandparents of the grandchild in terms of the definitions of these roles that each brings to the growing relationship.

Family sociologists have argued that the closeness and degree of relatedness of kin may influence the amount of interaction between them, but the closeness or degree of relatedness is based on an assumption that those concerned are aware of the relationship. Certainly we are accustomed to distinguish first cousins who we may interact with fairly frequently at times from second cousins who are seen rarely. Most people are able easily to describe their relations, indicating the closeness of interest, feeling and intimacy, as well as distinguishing the degree of the relatedness, and in so doing assume that such kinship relationships have some meaning for them, acknowledging rights, obligations and expectations which are implicit in the relationship. Even the word 'relation' is an indication of the special nature of the relationship which marks it off from those of 'neighbour' or 'friend'. In fact kinsfolk can feel hurt and dismayed if these special expectations are not fulfilled. What we are saying is that some relatives are deceived by other relatives and that in a society which sets great store by such virtues as integrity, honesty and truthfulness AID is totally inconsistent with these values as long as secrecy is essential to the process.

Until recently it has been accepted without question by most medical practitioners writing about their experience of AID that the best course of action for the infertile couple was to keep the fact of AID secret and to allow relatives, friends and the child to assume that the conception was 'natural'. Indeed this has been seen as one of the advantages of AID when compared to the other alternative that may be available to the infertile couple, namely, adoption. Therefore, whilst awareness that the child was conceived by AID is restricted, the expectations of kin will be no different from those in a normal family. No one but the parents and the AID practitioner need know that a particular child was conceived by AID. But the basis of these family relationships is being artificially supported by the maintenance of this secret over a long period of time, indeed, often for life. Relatives, therefore, who are not party to the secret and who assume normal blood ties with the child have expectations with respect to rights and obligations towards the child, which are based on a false premiss: a false premiss which is known to be false by *some* members of the kin network (the child's mother and her husband), but not others. This is not to say that if these kin were aware of the AID background they would necessarily reject the child. It is of interest to notice that if there is no secret there may be a differential reaction to the child by kinsfolk in that it is possible that knowledge of the husband's sterility will mean less to the mother's kin than to the husband's kin for blood ties with the AID child will still be present for the former.

If the secret is kept it is reasonable to suppose that keeping it for a long time from one's kin may produce stress for an AID couple. Such stress may increase over time, for as the child grows older and begins to ask, what in other children, would be regarded as innocent questions about his or her origins, the AID secret may become progressively more difficult to keep.

It may be asked: why do the AID couple not tell their close kin and especially their parents? Certainly the evidence shows that many find this to be impossible. In times past adoptions were kept secret, yet today in our own society it is held highly desirable to tell the child he is adopted and not unduly to conceal the fact from others. But of course, in adoption, the parents and other close kin of the couple invariably know the child has been adopted. The arguments supporting openness are not based on a belief that it is easy to do, but rather it is held that an atmosphere created by secrecy and deceit is even harder to bear and may well provide an ambience conducive to more serious problems for both the adopted child and the family of which he has become a part. Indeed, some advocate openness on the grounds that concealment consumes so much emotional energy that could be better expended in a more creative manner in dealing with the problems that knowledge entails. The fact is, however, that many AID couples find it next to impossible to reveal their decision to undergo AID to families and friends. R. T. Francoeur, who favours 'new trends in human reproduction', also recognises this in his book *Utopian Motherhood, New Trends in Human Reproduction* (1970) when he points out that even educated couples find it 'psychologically and emotionally difficult to cope with the reality and implications of artificial insemination' (p. 20).

Yet, if it is impossible to tell parents, either because the couple are afraid of the reaction or because they fear the secret cannot be shared by any larger number of people, then concealment must in some way affect the relationship between the AID couple and their parents. It is not a case of information being revealed which has no relevance to the relationship; quite the contrary, for with the best will in the world, and with compassion and understanding together with a willingness to accept the child, as adopted children are accepted by the wider kinsfolk of the couple, there remains the fact that the child is not biologically related to one set of kin. Those who are not related by blood, the husband's kin, are bound to look on the child, if not personally, then socially, as different from those who are biologically related. To conceal the nature of the child's own conception therefore is to persist in maintaining a deception; a deception that cannot be overlooked or easily forgotten because it introduces a false assumption into the relationship between the kin who are kept in ignorance and the knowing couple.

Again we ask 'for whom is AID being kept secret?'. What makes keeping the AID secret from close kin so desirable? Is it *really* to protect the child from the painful discovery that his social father (pater) is not his biological father (genitor), and from the subsequent problems of self-identity to which this may give rise? Or is secrecy maintained in order to protect the husband's feelings in his attempt to appear normal by having children as other husbands do? There is, however, another factor and one not to be taken lightly. This concerns the current legal situation, for whilst AID is not illegal in itself it leads to a situation for which there is no legal provision and at the present time in the UK and some other countries there is no legal way of registering an AID birth. This has implications for inheritance. Thus one AID couple, highly intelligent and able people, who voluntarily approached the authors with information about themselves, were willing for friends to know and had, in fact, told the wife's mother, but faced a legal difficulty because the husband was divorced from his first wife who had had children by him. Should she know of his present situation she might take steps to see that the AID child did not inherit after his death, so that her own children might be the better provided for. In his case he had had an irreversible vasectomy, the irreversibility having been concealed. It will be appreciated that the sources of guilt in connection with secrecy about AID may be legion, not merely restricted to interpersonal relationships with grandparents and other close kin but also extending to other children and former spouses.

There is yet another reason why the AID family may be driven to conceal its nature. This is the stigma which may attach itself to the family as a whole and not just to the child. Even if the law were changed in order to legitimise the AID child in some way, it is unlikely the stigmatisation associated with illegitimate reproduction would disappear entirely, at least not immediately. Despite such a legal change the oddity of the practice of AID would remain in the public mind. As D. Gill points out in his book *Illegitimacy, Sexuality and the Status of Women*, the prevailing attitude is that children need, and ought, to be reared in a complete family unit. Stigmatisation of children known to have been conceived 'unnaturally' is unlikely to disappear entirely from the Western social scene in the immediate future. Such stigmatisation may well lead to a sense of deprivation. In the case of the mother of an illegitimate child she may find it very difficult to hide the result of her conception and pregnancy, but the mother of an AID child will not have this difficulty provided her husband's infertility or impotency is kept secret, and kept secret from not only wider kinsfolk, and the kin of orientation (i.e. his and her parents and their siblings and siblings' children), but even within the AID family itself. Yet whilst it may be easier in this respect to keep the AID secret there are other respects which make keeping the secret very difficult without incurring stress of some kind.

At this point we enter an area of great ignorance and we can but speculate. J. Holland, in her article 'Adoption and artificial insemination: some implications' (1971), says 'it is doubtful that people can really live in intimate relation to each other without revealing at least some part of their emotionally charged secret knowledge or without being significantly affected by the necessity for keeping it'. And she goes on: 'if the child does eventually discover the truth, the fact that it was such a dark secret will make him assume that there is something "wrong" about it . . . and therefore about him." She also quotes V. Bernard as saying that the problem is not so much that one parent may blurt out the truth but rather 'at a subtler level, the young child's partial overhearing of mysterious allusions, and his sensing of parental lies, half-truths and evasions may incur confusion, suspicion and anxiety for which he needs his parent's help – instead, he feels cut off from them by a conspiracy of silence'. Indeed, children who are believed to have been kept in ignorance are often aware of some mystery surrounding them. This may well result in a distortion of the truth leading to quite fantastic beliefs. As mentioned in Chapter 4, in one instance the children were of the opinion they were the result of virgin births. The fact of their being different from other children may be less harmful than the consequence of the distorted self-images they may conjure up.

Stress is also likely to increase if the secret is perceived to be in danger because it is shared with others. As Benjamin Franklin said, 'If you would keep your secret from an enemy tell it not to a friend'. And there is some reason for such cynicism. Two people may keep a secret but it is seldom that three can. This is because telling a secret is a means of establishing a closer relationship with the one to whom it is revealed. Moreover, whilst a secret may be kept by one person for some days, length of time appears to weaken the resolve not to share it with a third person. In fact secrets are for telling! Thus, should the AID couple reveal their secret to one other person, a parent or friend or neighbour, it is likely that before long others will know. Their secret shared with the AI practitioner is as safe as his administrative machinery is secure and his professional code strongly held to, and in most cases doubtless confidentiality is maintained, but beyond this there is great uncertainty. For example, if an AID mother re-married would she keep the secret from her second husband or share it with him, and if a child is born of this second marriage will she keep it from that child? What is likely to happen in the event of a divorce when the husband marries again and has to explain his sterility in the face of the fact that he ostensibly is the genitor of a child by his previous marriage?

If with regard to the AID family's secret we can only speculate about the degree of stress engendered and the risks of disclosure that are present, we can say something in general about the social implications of secrecy. It was the German sociologist Georg Simmel, writing before the First World War, who in his essay *The Secret and the Secret Society* made the point that in the modern world, as contrasted with the primitive or traditional society, life is based to a much larger extent than is usually realised upon faith in the honesty of others. This is so in the economy, which depends so much on credit, or in science, where researchers rely on the integrity of each other in their employment of methods of inquiry. Thus the lie becomes something much more devastating than in an earlier age. 'If the few persons closest to us lie, life becomes unbearable', he observed, but it is also true that whilst ethically negative, a lie can, so long as it is not revealed, be a factor of quite positive sociological significance for the formation of a relationship. Indeed, if one party has some guilty secret in relation to another it may well cause him or her to exhibit a considerateness, a delicacy of manner, a wish to make up for the guilt feelings by being more than normally selfless, which would not be there if he had no troubled conscience. This is why we may be inclined to consider the AID couple to be especially careful in their behaviour towards each other and towards their AID child.

The sociology of secrecy is not without its interest in relation to the family. We have all heard of 'family secrets', but let us consider the kinds of relationships in which the secret plays a part. Marriage is of two people, a marriage of 'true minds' as well as two bodies. It is as Simmel says a *dyad*, a group of two persons, who interact and who share a unique knowledge which no other person shares.

The fact is that there is a difference between a dyadic group and any larger group. This consists in the fact that 'the dyad has a different relation to each of its two elements than have larger groups to *their* members'. The point Simmel makes, and it is an important point, is that the group of two does not attain a super-personal status. In a group of two, were one to die, the group would disappear. In the case of a group of three or more the group survives the death of one member; it is super-personal. This we can see whenever the AID family splits up, and on divorce one partner marries again. But it can happen when the secret the AID couple share is shared with *any* third person.

We have raised the twin issues of strain and stress entailed in maintaining secrecy about AID but how may we go about discussing these in the AID family? R. Hill has developed a theoretical framework for analysing stress in families in general which may help us. Briefly, he suggests there are four factors: the husband and wife face a situation where the critical event (A) interacts with the resources the family possesses for meeting crises (B) and these in turn interact with the way the family interprets the event (C) to produce the crisis itself (X). Now (B) and (C) lie within the family which we may describe in terms of certain relationship structures and values, but (A) is outside the family. Hill calls (A) the *stressor event* and clearly in the AID family the exposure of the secret is such a stressor event, and it will vary in degree. If a very close relative or friend comes to learn the truth of the AID birth it may be much less of a threat than if a garrulous neighbour comes by it. Again, it will depend on the degree to which (B) represents the family's vulnerability. Of course, we may expect that where the stressor event is sudden or unexpected its disruptive force will be greater. This is why adoptive parents are counselled to tell the child at as early a date as possible of his adoption and to repeat it at intervals as the child gets older. In AID it is much more difficult to discuss the subject with a young child. This is clearly demonstrated by our correspondent in her letter reproduced in Chapter 4.

Vulnerability to stress may vary greatly from one family to another. It will be dependent on the degree to which the family is integrated, both within itself as a two-generation nuclear family, and also as a larger kinship unit. It will depend on the degree to which members of the family are adaptable to changing circumstances and here we may well have great variations according to the way the wife and her husband have been brought up and indeed the way they have reared their AID child. The personal influences of the various actors may well be a factor of importance and the degree of courage, fortitude, imagination and sensitivity they have to each other will all play their part. Finally, there is the position of people in the group and its influence. All this makes it very hard to generalise but it does perhaps indicate to us the kinds of consideration we have to bear in mind where family stress is concerned.

Let us at this point make it clear that stress is of two kinds. First, there is the strain and stress of maintaining a secret over a lengthy period of time. Secondly, there is the stress arising from a sudden disclosure of the secret; a possibility always present which may become more acute with time. There is some evidence that marriages that seem to be strong, and where there is a close understanding between the partners, are enriched by the acquisition of an AID child. This may be because the strain and stress of keeping a secret are contained by such a good relationship. But this does not mean that the family will be able to withstand the shock of sudden exposure. The stressor event may be a long-term background worry but it may also be a sudden thunderbolt out of the blue. The tragedy for the AID family is that both are present. Hill in his treatment of the subject theoretically is concerned with the sudden crisis; the sociology of the family has not devoted itself to long-term stress and so we must look elsewhere for an understanding of this problem.

Yet however much we argue in favour of the AID family keeping its secret and coping with the strains and stresses the secret engenders, there is the wider society to consider, for the society is greater than the family, the neighbourhood, or the local community. We have already indicated how modern society depends on trust and confidence which enables so many social processes to operate, processes such as the banking system, the stock exchange, the professions, and so forth. But trust is also essential for the existence of family and kinship relationships. It is for this reason that AID is a practice which society cannot at present unequivocally approve. This is reflected in the inconsistency in our social norms. Indeed, English society is in a state of confusion, for whilst the law maintains that the AID child is illegitimate the national health service provides a means of obtaining AID. We may well ask: is it not time the practice of AID was made legal and the stigma of illegitimacy removed from the child? Can we not have a new category: a register of 'accepted children' or a new status such as 'semi-adoption', or indeed plainly 'AID children', if we must preserve something of the legitimate status of children born in wedlock?

The answer to this question is not easy to determine. The problem may be a legal one but there are extra-legal aspects. Indeed, the problem is not so much a matter of legislative change as of the attitudes of people. To what degree would new legal provision be used? How could it be enforced? If the stigma is not to be removed completely then people will be unlikely to avail themselves of new legal provisions; it is by no means certain legal provision can or will remove the stigma. Moreover, if there is built into the registration of births some uncertainty, an indeterminacy about the status of a family and the children of that family, will not the entire institutional structure of marriage and family life be threatened? Of course, it may be pointed out that there have been many changes in recent years; attitudes in particular are different in many respects today from those of a few decades ago. There is more sympathy for the unmarried mother, and there is more tolerance for cohabiting people who are not married. But this does not mean that for the vast majority of people the institution of marriage is unimportant, or is less important than formerly. What has to be said is that for those who adhere to the traditional norms, the structure of family relationships depends for its existence on nothing less than confidence; confidence that what is declared to be the case is in fact the case. In short the family depends for its existence on trust. Remove this basis for integrity and not only marriage and family life, but social stability is threatened at its very foundation.

We may ask if modern society can allow the present situation to continue. To be sure it may do so provided AID is responsible for a minute proportion of births, provided professional people restrict it to suitable couples and that it does not proliferate. Unfortunately these and other assumptions are unsound, as we shall show in the next chapter.

Can we then suppress AID ? Surely not, for the technique is a simple one and becomes simpler, the practice is covert and easy. The fact is that the problem is not only unsolved but it appears to be insoluble.

We have in this chapter traced the problem of secrecy in AID from within the AID family itself through wider kinship links to the society as a whole, and it would appear we have come to no clear conclusion, but then we did not expect to. What we hope to have revealed is the threat AID may entail for normal family life, a point made in the Feversham Report in 1960. Before passing on to the next chapter, however, it may be worth pausing to consider the matter from another angle, namely, that of the donor and his family, who are also part of our society.

The Feversham Report recommended that a married donor should obtain his wife's consent to what he does. We ask, why limit this to his wife? If a donor is not married why not obtain his fiancée's consent, and if unmarried and with no fiancée, what of any future wife he may marry; has she no 'rights' in this matter and what of children she may have by him? What rights, obligations and hence expectations do other members of his family have with respect to the children he is helping to be born? He, the donor, may not want to be a father, but his mother might wish to be a grandmother. In fact one mother of a donor in a television programme expressed concern at her ignorance of the number of her 'grandchildren' whom she believed were in existence somewhere.

We may put it bluntly and perhaps crudely, but surely pertinently: whose sperm is it? Who owns it? Is it satisfactory to say it is the donor's? In one sense it is, but a moment's reflection will show that in another, but very real sense, it is not entirely his to do as he wants with it. Thus, for example, we do not allow abortion on demand. A woman does not have an exclusive right to do what she wants with her body, so why should he? A person has no 'right' to commit suicide, and until fairly recently it was a crime to do so. The fact is that society does not permit us to do what we like with our bodies for the simple reason that we are part of society. 'No man is an island entire of itself'. No one is a complete individual apart from society. We all belong to each other.

Finally, let us note that in considering, as we have in this chapter, the nature of paternity, and what it means to be a relative, we have begun through a consideration of AID to come closer to an understanding of the normal family, a subject on which a great deal more remains to be said.

6

Implications and Conclusions

Up until this point we have assumed that AID is taking place within a family consisting of a sterile husband and his wife. Indeed, all the major reports on AID have also been based on this assumption. Had it been otherwise the recommendations of the Feversham and Peel committees would probably have been different, and the Archbishop of Canterbury's commission would very likely have been even more forceful in its condemnation of the practice. Whilst AID was a procedure affecting a tiny minority and whilst its provision could be contained by the medical profession, there was little reason for the state to interfere. The Feversham Committee may be criticised because it failed to make positive recommendations or proposals for the regulation of AID, preferring merely not to encourage the practice. This committee believed that public recognition of AID would probably lead to an increase in its use and that its regulation would create more problems than the practice does. In its view discouragement of the practice was preferable to its condemnation, an attitude adopted by the Archbishop's commission twelve years earlier.

In recent years several important developments have taken place, and had the Feversham Committee had the foresight to see these developments it would probably not have been so complacent in its inaction. Thus an opportunity was missed to provide guidance from a broadly based committee which could be said to represent the community as a whole which left it to a more narrowly based medical 'panel' to make positive recommendations. As a result of the acceptance of the recommendation of the Peel Committee that AID centres should be opened within the national health service, the practice of AID is no longer a matter of slight importance serving a small minority of people by a few medical practitioners out of public sight. Feversham argued that the practice was a matter between individual couples and their medical advisers; formally to make statements about it (whether to promote or condemn it) was to recognise its social importance which in turn implied a policy position of some kind. That committee felt it was wise to keep the subject where it belonged, in the private doctor's surgery where the atmosphere was one of confidentiality and discretion. However, the Peel Committee, by suggesting the introduction of AID into the national health service, extended the provision of AID from what was a purely private medical matter to one of public policy. By trying, doubtless with the best of possible motives, to provide what it thought to be a medical service to people in need, the Peel Committee effectively opened the topic of AID to debate in a way that the Feversham Committee had tried to avoid.

It may be asked: why should this issue of AID be of concern today? Why is it necessary to open the Pandora's box where until now deception, secrecy, anonymity and confidentiality have lain dormant and unobserved? By their exposure the dangers of recrimination, guilt and the creation of stress for the four participants and the child are increased. Why should such risks be greater now than before the Peel and Feversham committees reported? The answer lies in three main developments that have taken place in recent years.

First, there is an increase in the number of people who are both aware of AID and are availing themselves of it. We noted in Chapter 1 that it had been estimated that about 1,500 couples each year, where the husband is found to be sterile, may actively consider recourse to AID. In addition some husbands who suffer from hereditary disease or have rhesus incompatibility with their wives may also seek AID. Whilst this incidence fixes a natural ceiling on the potential number of AID couples, the practice could be thought to be relatively rare. However, this figure is no longer a realistic one when vasectomy, divorce and re-marriage are taken into consideration. An increasing number of couples requesting AID are married for the second time after the husband has undergone a vasectomy following the birth of the children of his first marriage. This negates previous attempts to measure the incidence of AID within the general population. In addition, we should take note of the current practice of providing AID for single girls and lesbian couples. In a society where there is a movement which stresses the woman's right to choose, this demand is likely to grow. We shall return to this issue later but it should be realised that the inclusion of vasectomised men, lesbian couples and single women as potential, and actual, users of AID makes nonsense of the previously accepted belief that the number of AID users will always be restricted to a small group.

Secondly, the provision outlets for AID have dramatically increased in recent years, both inside and outside the national health service. We do not know the total number of such outlets but the AID outlets alone are known to be in excess of three dozen. The lack of information about both the total number of AID users and the number of AID provision centres is the result of the secrecy surrounding the practice. Apparently, no one can provide these figures with any precision; at best, the figures that are given can only be the result of guesswork.

Thirdly, the techniques employed in the provision of AID

have been simplified. There was a time when the only way a woman could obtain AID was by attending a particular place at which the donor's semen would be delivered at the right time. Today doctors are not the only ones with access to semen and the technique no longer requires a medically qualified person in the way once thought necessary.

These three developments mean that we are in a very different situation from that which faced the Feversham Committee. This being so the chances of the misuse of AID are likely to be increased.

AID is just one aspect of a new technology in reproduction and cannot be considered in isolation. If the Feversham Report advised against control it did so in the situation as it was in 1960, but time has marched on, technology has developed and, what is much more important perhaps, attitudes among a section of the population have changed. We cannot go back to the 1960s. Indeed, once the state took cognisance of AID by acting on the recommendations of the Peel Committee of the British Medical Association it was clear that it was no longer possible to assume that AID could be discouraged, or at least remain a process about which most people were in ignorance. The question arises: how much more control can there be and with what ultimate effect on our society? Is control of this and other aspects of reproduction an escalating process? Here is a subject for public debate.

The work of Patrick Steptoe and Robert Edwards in fertilising an ovum outside the mother's body and then replanting it in her womb, leading to the first successful birth of a child by this means, is but a beginning. We are now told that cryobiologists are at present conducting experiments to deep-freeze human embryos in their early genesis to hold them in a state of suspended animation for months or even years, eventually to be thawed and implanted in the reproductive tract of *another* woman for normal birth; a child conceived today might well be born in a hundred years' time!

But this apart, it is presumably now possible to envisage the surrogate mother of another's baby: a woman may have a child *of her own* without having to endure the gestation period, by a man who may, or may not, be her husband, or even known to her. Here, if ever, is the possibility of dispensing with the family as we know it today. Such a process as this is possible, for already the practice has been employed in relation to agricultural stock. We are not then in the realm of science fiction but of possible realities. What kinds of decision-making are entailed in such processes, and who makes the decisions? Are we to have a state apparatus to do it? Is it to be left to the medical profession, and if so will there be a consistent policy? Is it a purely medical matter anyway? How can officialdom be so controlled that it will not use these techniques for its own ends to the possible destruction of human freedom and the family?

Alternatively, absence of control over AID means that increasingly it will become a private enterprise. This means that in the absence of an agreed code of practice different policies will be pursued by different people and organisations. The first area where this will be manifested is in the selection of people for AID. We have already seen that some couples who have been deemed unsuitable to receive a child for adoption may be favourably considered for AID. In fact, it may well be that AID may be had on demand. In recent years publicity has been given to lesbian 'couples' who desire a child; and mention has already been made of the gynaecologist who was willing to perform this service. Indeed one national newspaper went on to declare that he had been 'responsible for the birth of ten babies to established lesbian couples both in Britain and abroad'. In 1979 the British Medical Association recognised that such activities were being carried on by members of its own profession but felt that the decision whether or not to undertake them was entirely at the discretion of the doctor and patient involved. Neither the BMA nor the Department of

Health intended to provide any guidelines concerning AID. An organisation known as Sappho, based in London, is known to have referred lesbians to a gynaecologist willing to provide an AID service, but others in the medical profession refuse to provide AID for such people. A representative of the Royal College of Obstetricians and Gynaecologists has observed that 'if donors knew their sperm was going to lesbians, one can't help wondering if they would think this was a good thing'.

There is, however, another group to be considered. These are single women, not necessarily lesbians, who wish to remain single yet also want to have a child of their own. Very often these are women of intelligence and ability, who wish to pursue a career. It may be argued that women generally today have a number of goals; to pursue a career, to have a child and to be happily married. For some the first two goals take precedence over the third. Indeed, it is the restrictions resulting from having a man about which concern them. The absence of a husband means such a woman can avoid male superiority, however that manifests itself. It means she can be geographically mobile in pursuing her career, it enables her to manage her own affairs single-mindedly without having to consider another's interests, and she may feel freer to raise a child of her own in the way she wishes. This is not the place to moralise on the use of AID for such a woman; what is important is to establish that it can happen, is likely to do so, and indeed has already taken place. If it is said that few would wish to adopt this policy and practice then we may point to the changing attitudes of recent times which for some women make liberation from male dominance a matter of great personal concern. In addition to this there may be a general maternal desire in women and these freer attitudes may permit them to have greater expression; certainly there are also cultural values in our society conferring considerable status on motherhood. Thus there is the attitude that a woman cannot experience a sense of fulfilment unless she has a child. Moreover, a child can be cared for by others, nursemaids, nursery schools, housekeepers, and so forth, to enable a single woman to achieve her maternal ambition as well as to pursue a career; a career which may well be financially rewarding enough to enable her to pay for these services. Thus AID could become a means of dispensing with marriage and the inconvenience of a husband and, of course, with a father too.

Before leaving the subject of AID for single women and lesbian couples let us briefly take up a point referred to in Chapter 5. This concerns keeping secret the origins of conception of the child. It appears that most couples with an AID child are not only reluctant to inform their parents and siblings, but also their friends and neighbours. In the case of single women and lesbian couples the secret can hardly be kept and therefore the practice is going to be more widely known. This being so we may well wonder what effect it will have on children in normal families. Will this not be an additional stimulus to children to question their own origins? Can they be certain they are the children of their parents? If this is the case then anxiety and uncertainty are injected into family life which has, until now, been contained. The teenage daughter of one of the authors, having overheard conversations about AID during the writing of this book, discreetly enquired of her mother if she herself was an AID baby!

We conclude then that in the absence of a clear and agreed code of practice all kinds of people may be accepted for AID, but in addition we have to ask ourselves a question about the supply of as well as the demand for donated semen. Thus the advent of new technology has made it possible to widen the basis of selection of donors, or perhaps in some cases we should call them vendors. Recent press publicity has focused on the California businessman who is reported as hoping to produce a super-race by inseminating high-IQ women with semen donated by Nobel Prize-winners. It was said that he intended to set up a sperm bank. The notion of a sperm bank appears to have originated some forty years ago in a proposal by H. J. Muller, an American geneticist who also won a Nobel Prize in the 1940s for discovering that radiation is harmful to human genes. Dr G. J. Annas writing in the *Hastings Center Report* (1979), says that two commercial sperm banks in the USA fill over a hundred orders a month, and one is preparing to market semen directly to consumers.

This kind of development, under no control but subject to commercial conditions, means that if the organisation can secure semen from certain kinds of people, be they donors or vendors, then there is a strengthening of those forces in society which stimulate demand. One can envisage football players and athletes being approached to produce semen in the interests of producing babies possessing outstanding physique. Indeed, all kinds of amateur eugenics can be envisaged on the part of suppliers and consumers. Already the home artificial insemination do-it-yourself kit is a possibility, maybe a reality. In a *Man Alive* programme broadcast on 21 November 1979 on BBC2 a respondent recorded how on a girl's ovulation day her friend had used a syringe to insert semen produced by a man known to them with a view to furnishing that man and his wife with a child they could not have had themselves. Certainly, with simplification of techniques and a commercial interest in making the practice of AID available to more and more people, the likelihood is for it to increase.

It is not difficult to see how the process may become fashionable in some quarters, with attendant risks for the normal family and society at large. The fact is that we are in a dilemma. On the one hand there is the danger of proliferation and uncontrolled commercialism with all the risks this has for normal practice, whilst on the other hand to regulate officially the practice both drives some practice underground and at the same time also undermines the institution of marriage and family life by its implications. As we have pointed out in Chapter 5, the state is involved in the provision of AID, and this creates doubt about legitimacy and connives at what may be variously regarded by some as a mild subterfuge and by others as the crime of perjury. The only way of dealing with this is to seize the horns of the dilemma and face the implications of AID.

CONCLUSIONS

Let us briefly consider where this discussion of the artificial family has led us.

AID may be said to have acquired respectability in so far as it tries to help those who have a personal need arising out of their childlessness. That it occurs in a clinical environment with the assistance of professional people adds to this respectability. It is a process which is not undertaken lightly. We hope we have amply demonstrated that AID may well benefit some couples who are childless and who are distressed by their childlessness. Moreoover, it may benefit them despite the strains and stresses AID may entail as a process, as a covert practice and as a continuing subterfuge. However, we have found it necessary to indicate that in so far as AID may be a threat to normal families and may arouse uncertainty in children's minds about their origins, and most particularly in so far as it usually does entail secrecy, it is undermining the social values of openness, honesty and truthfulness on which social institutions and the institutional behaviour we know as family life rests.

Whilst not denying that some couples may have been enriched by having children through AID we can understand the view of the Feversham Committee that AID should not be encouraged and we see some reason for this arising from a sociological analysis of its effects on society at large and the normative order which upholds it. By giving some recognition to AID through national health service provision, we have as a nation placed ourselves in a contradictory position, for the government is providing a service with no legal base, AID not being recognised in law and the AID child only legitimate if adopted. How long the nation can continue to ignore AID whilst providing a service that in most cases leads to husbands breaking the law and couples maintaining a conspiracy of silence, and whilst at the same time some single women and lesbian couples have recourse to it openly, and sometimes defiantly, is not for us to say. However, we point to an increasing occurrence of the practice and to increasing publicity about it.

It would appear that attitudes on the part of AID practitioners and among the medical profession are varied, sometimes varying very considerably. Indeed, many statements which have been made from time to time appear to us to be inconsistent, ambiguous and sometimes contradictory and this seems to arise because there is no well-defined framework within which practitioners can work. Perceptions of practitioners differ accordingly as they consider people's needs. Thus some practitioners are willing to provide AID for single women whilst others abhor the idea. What some regard as a matter for confidentiality and clinical judgement others may regard as deceit and idiosyncratic thoughtlessness. It is here that the difficulty of introducing some regulation into the provision of AID rests, for whether the behaviour of AI practitioners is approved or not by individual members of their own profession, most doctors believe that decisions concerning AID are a matter solely between the AI practitioner and the AID couple. In other words, the sanctity of the freedom of clinical judgement and the confidentiality which this implies are paramount.

Nevertheless, there are boundaries within which such clinical freedom can be exercised. Besides the professional regulation of a doctor's conduct, society also places restrictions on the clinical freedom of medical practitioners. In the case of abortion, for instance, there is a clear legal framework imposed by the state which the doctor must not contravene.

In the absence of a socially approved framework for the provision of AID, a very heavy responsibility is being placed upon individual medical practitioners. A close examination of AID reveals that in the absence of external guidance a reliance on clinical judgement is far from comfortable. For example, the doctor is usually 'treating' the fit wife of the sterile husband. Perhaps it is for this reason that emphasis is often made on treating the AID couple rather than an individual. Again, AID is not concerned with the preservation of life but with its creation. In the case of a fertile woman receiving AID even the need for the expertise of a medically qualified person may be questioned.

One difficulty in obtaining more open debate about the practice of AID is that many practitioners feel that the whole subject is a matter of clinical judgement on their part based on the confidentiality that they feel they are professionally required to maintain between themselves and the AID couple. In this book we have attempted to show that AID is a subject that is far more complex than this. We accept that there is an undoubted area of medical confidentiality and clinical freedom within the AID relationships described, but by claiming the need for confidentiality covering the whole topic of AID provision, effective discussion about the practice is being hampered. We see a distinction between the confidentiality existing between the AI practitioner and the AID couple, the anonymity of the donor and the secrecy existing within the AID family, between that family and wider kin and in relation to society as a whole. Whilst we accept the professional limitation on open discussion of the confidential nature of the first of these relationships, the same rules do not apply in relation to anonymity and secrecy. Those outside the medical profession have not only a right but a duty to debate the issues of anonymity and secrecy which affect society as a whole.

It follows that what are required are such regulations as are deemed necessary and a professional code of practice. The chief questions which arise are: what should be their content and who should be responsible for determining them? We strongly suggest that AID is not merely a medical matter but also one of social and hence moral and legal concern.

To be more precise, we argue for a governmental initiative to set up a suitable body to examine the situation. It should be widely representative of society and not restricted to a medical and administrative membership. AID is primarily a social matter and not just a medical one. Therefore legal, religious and educational interests as well as medical issues should be represented, together with some technical guidance from social scientists.

To make a start we list below those questions which we believe should be taken into account. In general terms consideration should be given to the kinds of control required, how they can be instituted with some expectation of success, and with what safeguards against misuse. Moreover, important aspects of human society such as general family welfare, the role of marriage in society and the well-being of children need to be included. The tasks facing such a body are therefore not inconsiderable; it would have to go over much of the ground the Feversham Committee covered, but as we have pointed out this would be justified by the developments that have taken place since that committee reported. The following appear to us to be among the questions to be considered:

THE CHILD

For whose benefit is AID undertaken – the child's or the couple's?

Does a child have a right to knowledge about his or her origins?

Are there dangers inherent in telling a child of his or her AID status?

Are there dangers inherent in attempting to keep AID a secret from the child?

Should AID parents be obliged to adopt the child?

Should there be legal changes in order to make the AID child legitimate?

What effect would legitimising AID children have on the status of children in normal families?

Should laws of inheritance be altered in favour of AID children?

What provision should be made for AID children in cases of divorce and separation?

Should follow-up inquiries of AID children be encouraged?

RECIPIENTS

What should be the criteria for selection?

Are the selection criteria amenable to assessment?

Who should be responsible for selection?

Should recipients be required to give written consent?

What is the effect of AID on the marital relationship of the AID couple?

What is the effect of denying AID on the marital relationship of the childless couple?

Does a woman who wants a baby have a right to one?

Should AID be available to lesbian women?

Should AID be available to single women?

What implications does the practice of vasectomy have for the practice of AID?

Should the AID father be deemed to be the legal father of the child?

THE AID KIN

Does secrecy have harmful effects on relationships within the wider AID family?

Should the relationships within the wider AID family be the subject of follow-up inquiry?

Do relatives of the AID child and couple have a right to knowledge about the child's origin?

THE DONOR

What should be the criteria for selection?

Are the selection criteria amenable to assessment?

Should donors receive counselling?

Who should be responsible for selection?

Should the donor be required to give written consent?

Should donors receive payment?

How frequently should the same donor be used?

Should there be a restriction to the number of offspring from each donor?

Should the donor have any legal liabilities in respect of the child?

Does the donor have a right to do with his semen as he sees fit?

THE DONOR'S KIN

Do relatives of the donor have a right to knowledge of the donor's participation?

Does the donor's participation have an effect upon his own marriage and family relationships?

To what extent should the donor's family be considered in the selection of the donor?

THE AI PRACTITIONER

What skills are required in the provision of artificial insemination?

Who should provide an AID service?

Who gives AID advice and how is it disseminated?

Should a counselling facility be mandatory?

Should specific training for AI practitioners be introduced?

Should non-medical practitioners be prohibited from providing an AID service?

What records should be kept by the AI practitioner?

How can the confidentiality of AID records be assured?

Should AI practitioners be registered?

CONTEMPORARY SOCIETY

What is the extent of the practice of AID in this country and what are the likely future developments?

Should AID receive open (rather than tacit) official recognition?

How far is adoption a model for AID?

Should the availability of AID be publicised?

What is the likely effect of increasing AID use on the children of normal families?

Does AID constitute a danger to the institutions of marriage and the family?

Does the deception surrounding AID undermine the values of society?

Should eugenic considerations be made explicit?

Should there be a special register of AID children?

Should there be a centralised system for selecting donors and storing semen similar to that in use by the blood transfusion service?

Should commercial sperm banks be permitted, and if so under what conditions of regulation and control?

What effect would regulation of AID provision have on other bio-technical advances in the field of reproduction?

Can AID be regulated effectively?

Bibliography

Adams, B. N. (1968), *Kinship in an Urban Setting* (Chicago: Markham).

Alexander, N. J. and Kay, R. (1977), 'Antigenicity of frozen and fresh spermatozoa', *Fertility and Sterility,* vol. 28, no. 11, pp. 1234–7.

Annas, G. J. (1979), 'Artificial insemination: beyond the best interests of the donor, *Hastings Center Report,* vol. 9, no. 4, pp. 14–15.

Anonymous (a medical practitioner) (1958), 'Artificial insemination. A critical review', *Family Planning,* vol. 7, no 1.

Ansbacher, R. (1978), 'Artificial insemination with frozen spermatozoa', *Fertility and Sterility,* vol. 29, no. 4, pp. 375–9.

'A Practitioner' (1958), 'Artificial Insemination', *Lancet,* 24 May, pp. 118–19.

Banks, A. L. (1968), 'Aspects of adoption and artificial insemination', in Behrman and Kistner (1975).

Barrett, A. T. (1978), 'Co-ordinating an AID program', *Contemporary Obstetrics/Gynecology,* vol. 12, pp. 123–9.

Barton, M., Walker, K. and Weisner, B. P. (1945), 'Artificial insemination', *British Medical Journal,* vol. 1, pp. 40–3.

Beck, W. W. (1974), 'Artificial insemination and semen preservation', *Clinical Obstetrics and Gynaecology,* vol. 17, no. 4, pp. 115–25.

Becker, H. (1963), *Outsiders* (New York: Free Press).

Behrman, S. J. and Kistner, R. W. (1975), *Progress in Infertility* (Boston, Mass.: Little, Brown).

Bernard, V. W. (1963), 'Adoption', in Deutsh, A. and Fishman, H. (eds), *Encyclopedia of Mental Health,* vol. 1 (New York: Watts).

Blacker, C. P. (1957), 'Artificial insemination (donor)', *Eugenics Review,* vol. 48, no. 4, pp. 209–11.

Blank, R. H. (1979), 'Human genetic technology: some political implications', *Social Science Journal,* vol. 16, no. 3, pp. 1–20.

Bibliography

Blizzard, J. (1977), *Blizzard and the Holy Ghost* (London: Peter Owen).

Bok, S. (1978), 'Lying to children: the risks of paternalism', *Hastings Center Report,* vol. 8, no. 3, pp. 10–13.

Bott, E. (1971 2nd edition), *Family and Social Network* (London: Tavistock).

Boyd, R. (1966), 'Indications for and techniques of artificial insemination in man', *Excerpta Medica International Congress Series,* no. 133, pp. 855–6.

Brandon, J. (1979), 'Telling the AID child', *Adoption and Fostering,* vol. 95, no. 1, pp. 13–14.

Brandon, J. and Warner, J. (1977), 'AID and adoption: some comparisons', *British Journal of Social Work,* vol. 7, no. 3, pp. 335–42.

Brewer, C. (1978), 'Let lesbians have a fecund choice', *General Practitioner,* 20 January.

Brooke-Little, J. P. (Richmond Herald of Arms) (1976), letter to *The Times,* 7 July.

Buckingham, M. S. (1977), 'The treatment of male subfertility', *Fertility and Contraception,* vol. 1, no. 4, pp. 71–7.

Burr, W. R. (1973), *Theory Construction and the Sociology of the Family* (New York: Wiley Interscience).

Cary, W. (1948), 'Results of artificial insemination with an extra-marital specimen (semi-adoption)', *American Journal of Obstetrics and Gynaecology,* vol. 56, pp. 727–32.

Chong, A. P. and Taymor, M. L. (1975), 'Sixteen years experience with therapeutic donor insemination', *Fertility and Sterility,* vol. 26, no. 8, pp. 791–5.

CIO (1966), *Fatherless by Law?* (London: Church Information Office).

Clark, H. (1971), 'Fate, the "experts" and individual choice', *Soundings: An Interdisciplinary Journal,* vol. 50, no. 4, pp. 331–43.

Coleman, A. H. (1965), 'Artificial insemination', *Journal of the National Medical Association,* vol. 57, no. 4, pp. 331–2.

Cozby, P. (1973), 'Self disclosure – a literature review', *Psychological Bulletin,* vol. 79, pp. 73–91.

Creighton, P. (1977), *Artificial Insemination by Donor* (Toronto: Anglican Book Centre).

Cusine, D. J. (1975), 'AID and the law', *Journal of Medical Ethics*, vol. 1, pp. 39–41.

Cusine, D. J. (1979), 'Problems of status arising from human artificial insemination', *Eugenics Society Bulletin*, vol. 11, no. 2, pp. 49–56.

Davis, K. and Blake, J. (1956), 'Social structure and fertility: an analytical framework', *Economic Development and Cultural Change*, vol. 4 (April), pp. 211–35.

Dixon, R. E. and Buttram, V. C. (1976), 'Artificial insemination using donor semen: a review of 171 cases', *Fertility and Sterility*, vol. 27, no. 2, pp. 130–4.

Dunstan, G. R. (1973), 'Moral and social issues arising from AID', in Wolstenholme and Fitzsimons (1973).

Dunstan, G. R. (1975), 'Ethical aspects of donor insemination', *Journal of Medical Ethics*, vol. 1, pp. 42–4.

Dunstan, G. R. (1976), 'The law and ethics of AID', letter to *The Times*, 20 July.

Farris, E. and Garrison, M. (1954), 'Emotional impact of successful donor insemination', *Obstetrics and Gynaecology*, vol. 3 (January), pp. 19–20.

Feversham Committee (1960), *Report of the Departmental Committee on Human Artificial Insemination*, Cmnd 1105 (London: HMSO).

Fiumara, N. J. (1972), 'Transmission of gonorrhoea by artificial insemination', *British Journal of Venereal Diseases*, vol. 48, pp. 308–9.

Francoeur, R. T. (1970), *Utopian Motherhood, New Trends in Human Reproduction* (Garden City, NY: Doubleday).

Frankel, M. S. (1975), 'Cryobanking of human sperm', *Journal of Medical Ethics*, vol. 1, pp. 36–8.

Fried, C. (1973), 'Ethical issues in existing and emergency techniques for improving human fertility', in Wolstenholme and Fitzsimons (1973).

Friedman, S. (1977), 'Artificial donor insemination with frozen human semen', *Fertility and Sterility*, vol. 28, no. 11, pp. 1230–3.

Fuchs, K., Brandes, J. M. and Paldi, E. (1966), 'Enhancement of ovulation by chorigon for successful artificial insemination', *International Journal of Fertility*, vol. 11, no. 2, pp. 211–14.

Gerstel, G. (1963), 'A psychoanalytic view of artificial donor insemination', *American Journal of Psychotherapy*, vol. 17, pp. 64–77.

Gill, D. (1977), *Illegitimacy, Sexuality and the Status of Women* (Oxford: Blackwell).

Glazer, B. G. and Strauss, A. L. (1967), *The Discovery of Grounded Theory: Strategies for Qualitative Research* (Chicago: Aldine).

Goldenberg, R. L. and White, R. (1977), 'Artificial insemination', *Journal of Reproductive Medicine*, vol. 18, no. 3, pp. 149–54.

Goodhart, G. B. (1976), 'Law and ethics of AID', letter to *The Times*, 26 July.

Goss, D. A. (1975), 'Current status of artificial insemination with donor semen', *American Journal of Obstetrics and Gynaecology*, vol. 122, pp. 246–52.

Gregoire, A. T. and Mayer, R. C. (1965), 'The impregnators', *Fertility and Sterility*, vol. 16, no. 1, pp. 130–4.

Guttmacher, A. F. (1960), 'The role of artificial insemination in the treatment of sterility', *Obstetrical and Gynaecological Survey*, vol. 15, pp. 767–85.

Hansard, 16 March 1949, vol. 161, no. 50, cols 401–2.

Hansard, 26 February 1958, vol. 207, no. 39, cols 992–3.

Hansen, D. A. (1965), 'Personal and positional influence in formal groups: propositions and theory for research on family vulnerability to stress', *Social Forces*, vol. 44, pp. 202–10.

Hansen, D. A. and Hill, R. (1964), 'Families under stress' in *Handbook of Marriage and the Family* (Chicago: Rand McNally).

Hard, A. D. (1909a), 'Artificial Impregnation', *Medical World*, vol. 27, p. 163.

Hard, A. D. (1909b), letter in *Medical World*, vol. 27, p. 306.

Harrison, R. F. and Wynn-Williams, G. (1973), 'Human artificial insemination', *British Journal of Hospital Medicine*, vol. 9, pp. 760–2.

Hill, A. M. (1970), 'Experiences with artificial insemination', *Australia and New Zealand Journal of Obstetrics and Gynaecology*, vol. 10, pp. 112–14.

Hill, R. (1949), *Families Under Stress* (New York; Harper).

Hillix, W. A., Harari, H. and Mohr, D. A. (1979), 'Secrets', *Psychology Today* (September).

Holland, J. (1971), 'Adoption and artificial insemination: some social implications', *Soundings: An Interdisciplinary Journal*, vol. 50, no. 4, pp. 302–7.

Horne, H. W. (1975), 'Artificial insemination by donor: an issue of ethical and moral values', *New England Journal of Medicine*, vol. 293, no. 17, pp. 873–4.

Hughes, L. (1978), review of his work by Clare Dover, 'Satisfied parents go back for more AID', *Doctor*, 23 March.

Iizuka, R. *et al.* (1968), 'The physical and mental development of children born following artificial insemination', *International Journal of Fertility*, vol. 13, no. 1, pp. 24–32.

IPPF (1979), 'Medico-legal aspects of AID', *IPPF Medical Bulletin*, vol. 13, no. 1, pp. 1–2.

Jackson, M. (1953), 'Adoption or AID?', *Proceedings of the 1st World Congress on Fertility and Sterility*, New York, 25–31 May, pp. 506–10.

Jackson, M. (1955), 'A method of concentrating human spermatozoa for artificial insemination', *Journal of Family Welfare*, vol. 11, no. 1, pp. 14–18.

Jackson, M. and Richardson, D. (1977), 'The use of fresh and frozen semen and human AI', *Journal of Biosocial Science*, vol. 9, pp. 251–62.

Jones, A. and Bodmer, W. F. (1974), *Our Future Inheritance: Choice or Chance?* (London: Oxford University Press).

Kerr, M. (1958), *The People of Ship Street* (London: Routledge & Kegan Paul).

Kerr, M. G. and Rogers, C. (1975), 'Donor insemination', *Journal of Medical Ethics*, vol. 1, pp. 30–3.

Kleegman, S. J. and Kaufman, S. A. (1966), 'Therapeutic donor insemination' in *Infertility in Women*, (Oxford: Blackwell).

Klein, J. (1965), *Samples from English Cultures* (London: Routledge & Kegan Paul).

Kohane, E. S. *et al.* (1967), 'The use of HCG in delayed ovulation during artificial insemination', *Fertility and Sterility*, vol. 18, no. 5, pp. 593–7.

Laing, R. D. and Esterson, A. (1964), *Sanity, Madness and the Family* (London: Tavistock).

Bibliography

Langer, G., Lemberg, E. and Sharf, M. (1969), 'Artificial insemination: a study of 156 successful cases', *International Journal of Fertility*, vol. 14, pp. 232–40.

Ledward, R. S. and Symonds, E. M. (eds) (1976), *Donor Insemination – Your Questions Answered* (Nottingham: Nottinghamshire Area Health Authority, Teaching).

Ledward, R. S. *et al.* (1976), 'The establishment of a programme of artificial insemination by donor semen within the national health service', *British Journal of Obstetrics and Gynaecology*, vol. 83, pp. 917–20.

Ledward, R. S. *et al.* (1979), 'Social factors in patients for artificial insemination by donor (AID)', *Journal of Biosocial Science*, vol. 11, no. 4, pp. 473–9.

Levie, L. H. (1967), 'An enquiry into the psychological effects on parents of artificial insemination with donor semen', *Eugenics Review*, vol. 59, pp. 97–104.

Levie, L. H. (1972), 'Donor insemination in Holland', *World Medical Journal*, vol. 19, pp. 90–1.

Løveset, J. (1951), 'Artificial insemination: the attitude of patients in Norway', *Fertility and Sterility*, vol. 2, no. 5, pp. 415–29.

McLaren, A. (1973), 'Biological aspects of AID', in Wolstenholme and Fitzsimons (1973).

Marshall, J. (1971), 'AID: an occasion for creative law making', *Soundings: An Interdisciplinary Journal*, vol. 50, no. 4, pp. 325–30.

Matheson, G. W. *et al.* (1969), 'Frozen human semen for artificial insemination', *American Journal of Obstetrics and Gynaecology*, vol. 104, pp. 495–501.

Matteson, R. L. and Terranova, G. (1977), 'Social acceptance of new techniques of child conception', *Journal of Social Psychology*, vol. 101, pp. 225–9.

Memorandum by the Council of the Law Society (1959), 'The legal implications of artificial insemination', *Law Society Gazette* (August).

Menning, B. E. (1979), 'Counselling infertile couples', *Contemporary Obstetrics/Gynecology*, vol. 13, pp. 101–8.

Mitchell, G. D. and Snowden, R. (1980), 'Why AID is more than a medical issue', *World Medicine*, 8 March, pp. 85–7.

Moghissi, K. S. *et al.* (1977), 'Homologous artificial insemination: a reappraisal', *American Journal of Obstetrics and Gynaecology*, vol. 129, pp. 909–15.

Muller, H. J. (1963), 'Genetic progress by voluntarily conducted germinal choice', in Wolstenholme (1963).

Murphy, D. P. (1964), 'Donor insemination. A study of 511 prospective donors', *Fertility and Sterility*, vol. 15, no. 5, pp. 528–33.

Newton, J. R. (1978), 'Artificial insemination with frozen stored donor semen', *British Journal of Obstetrics and Gynaecology*, vol. 85, no. 9, pp. 641–4.

Newill, R. (1976), 'AID – a review of 200 cases', *British Journal of Urology*, vol. 48, pp. 139–44.

Norton, R., Feldman, C. and Tafoya, D. (1974), 'Risk parameters across types of secrets', *Journal of Counselling Psychology*, vol. 21, pp. 450–4.

Ostrom, K. (1971), 'Psychological considerations in evaluating AID', *Soundings: An Interdisciplinary Journal*, vol. 50, no. 4, pp. 290–301.

Payne, J. (1978), 'Talking about children: an examination of accounts about reproduction and family life', *Journal of Biosocial Science*, vol. 10, no. 4, pp. 367–74.

Peel Committee (1973), 'Report of the Panel on Human Artificial Insemination', *British Medical Journal*, 2, supplementary appendix V, p. 3.

Pennington, G. W. and Naik, S. (1977), 'Donor insemination: report of a two year study', *British Medical Journal*, vol. 1, pp. 1327–30.

Piattelli-Palmarini, M. (1973), 'Biological roots of the human individual, in Wolstenholme and Fitzsimons (1973).

Quinlivan, W. L. G. and Sullivan, H. (1977), 'Spermatozoal antibodies in human seminal plasma as a cause of failed artificial donor insemination', *Fertility and Sterility*, vol. 28, no. 10, pp. 1082–5.

Raboch, J. and Tomasek, Z. D. (1967), 'Therapeutic donor insemination – results', *Journal of Reproduction and Fertility*, vol. 14, pp. 421–5.

Ramsay, P. (1970), *Fabricated Man. The Ethics of Genetic Control* (New Haven, Conn.: Yale University Press).

Bibliography

RCOG (1976), *Artificial Insemination: Proceedings of the Fourth Study Group*, ed. M. Brudenell *et al.* (London: RCOG).

RCOG (1979a), 'Recommendations for centres planning to set up an AID service', leaflet.

RCOG (1979b), *Artificial Insemination*, explanatory information booklet for patients (London: RCOG).

Reiss, P. J. (1962), 'The extended kinship system: correlates of and attitudes on frequency of interaction', *Marriage and Family Living*, vol. 24, pp. 333–9.

Report of a Commission Appointed by His Grace the Archbishop of Canterbury (1948), *Artificial Human Insemination* (London: Society for the Propagation of Christian Knowledge).

Richards, R. P. (1971), 'Ethical and theological aspects', *Soundings: An Interdisciplinary Journal*, vol. 50, no. 4, pp. 315–23.

Rubin, B. (1965), 'Psychological aspects of human artificial insemination', *Archives of General Psychiatry*, vol. 13, pp. 121–32.

Sandler, B. (1965), 'Artificial insemination – the social implications', *Mental Health* (February).

Sandler, B. (1972), 'Donor insemination in England', *World Medicine*, vol. 19, pp. 87–9.

Schellen, A. (1957), *Artificial Insemination in the Human* (New York: Elsevier).

Schoysman, R. (1975), 'Problems of selecting donors for AI', *Journal of Medical Ethics*, vol. 1, pp. 34–5.

Sherman, J. K. (1964), 'Synopsis of the use of frozen human semen since 1964: state of the art of human semen banking', *Fertility and Sterility*, vol. 24, no. 5, pp. 397–412.

Simmel, G. (1950), *The Sociology of Georg Simmel*, trans. and ed. K. H. Wolff (Glencoe, Ill.: Free Press).

Simmons, F. A. (1957), 'The role of the husband in therapeutic donor insemination', *Fertility and Sterility*, vol. 8, no. 6, pp. 547–50.

Slome, J. (1973), 'Artificial insemination by donor', *British Medical Journal*, vol. 2, p. 365 (letter).

Snowden, R. and Mitchell, G. D. (1980), 'Anonymous AID for the childless couple', *New Scientist*, 13 March, pp. 828–9.

Stewart, W. (1954), 'What should the doctor know about

exogamous artificial insemination?', *Journal of American Medical Women's Association*, vol. 9, no. 11, pp. 368–70.

Stone, O. M. (1973), 'English law in relation to AID and embryo transfer', in Wolstenholme and Fitzsimons (1973).

Sulweski, J. M. *et al.* (1978), 'A longitudinal analysis of artificial insemination with donor semen', *Fertility and Sterility*, vol. 29, no. 5, pp. 527–31.

Teper, S. (1975), 'Social theory and individual fertility behaviour: some issues of research orientation', *Social Science and Medicine*, vol. 9, pp. 195–205.

Titmuss, R. M. (1971), *The Gift Relationship* (London: Allen & Unwin).

Triseliotis, J. (1973), *In Search of Origins: The Experiences of Adopted People* (London: Routledge & Kegan Paul).

Tyler, E. T. (1973), 'The clinical use of frozen semen banks', *Fertility and Sterility*, vol. 24, no. 5, pp. 413–16.

Valensin, G. (1960), *Artificial Insemination in Women* (London: Calder).

Veenhoven, R. (1975), 'Is there an innate need for children?', *European Journal of Social Psychology*, vol. 4, no. 4, pp. 495–501.

Wagner, A. (Garter King of Arms) (1976), letter to *The Times*, 26 July.

Warner, M. P. (1974), 'Artificial insemination. Review after thirty-two years experience', *New York State Journal of Medicine*, vol. 13, pp. 2358–61.

Watters, W. W. and Souza-Poza, J. (1966), 'Psychiatric aspects of artificial insemination (donor)', *Canadian Medical Association Journal*, vol. 95, no. 3, pp. 106–13.

Wolstenholme, G. E. W. (ed.) (1963) *Man and His Future*, CIBA Foundation Symposium (London: Churchill).

Wolstenholme, G. E. W. and Fitzsimons, D. W. (eds) (1973), *Law and Ethics of AID and Embryo Transfer*, CIBA Foundation Symposium 17 (N.S.) (Amsterdam: Associated Scientific Publishers).

Young, M. and Willmott, P. (1962), *Family and Kinship in East London* (Harmondsworth: Penguin).

Index

Index

Also published in Counterpoint

SOCIALISM IN A COLD CLIMATE

edited by John Griffith

"Thatcherism will leave two appalling legacies for the next Labour Government. One will be a crippled industrial base and the other will be a severely damaged welfare state. Never since 1945 will there have been so extensive a need for reconstruction. But the problems will, in one respect, be more severe than those created by six years of war. In 1945, Labour had some remedies to hand. Nationalisation of basic industries, the creation of a national health service, the replacement of the poor law, the establishment of social welfare, the relief of poverty, all these presented themselves as opportunities in a world where it was possible to make things new.

Tomorrow will not be the same. The Labour administrations of the sixties and the seventies provided very few fresh insights into the way socialism should develop in the eighties and nineties. The old Labourism will not do. The problems are different, the future is more dangerous, the structures of national and international society have changed."

This stimulating and important book is a thoughtful contribution to the considerable debate about the first steps to be taken to build a socialist society in the cold climate of the 1980s. It is not a handbook for immediate revolution or an instant blueprint for policy, nor does it assume that the remedies will be quick and easy – or orthodox. It is a book of ideas for the intelligent lay-person interested in politics and society whether of a socialist view or not. It covers topics as diverse as concepts of equality and fairness, sex discrimination, economic policy, health and urban policy, pensions, poverty and the economics of the welfare state, defense and internationalism.

Socialism in a Cold Climate will be essential and rewarding reading to all those interested in British politics, in the Labour party or in socialism generally.

THE INCREDIBLE EURODOLLAR
Or Why the World's Money System is Collapsing

W. P. Hogan and Ivor F. Pearce

The Eurodollar Market is an unprecedented phenomenon of awe-inspiring dimensions. It deals in accumulated international debt currently totalling US$1,300,000,000,000, a figure of the order of three times the entire stock of money in U.S.A., not too much less than the whole of that country's gross national product. If present trends continue, and there is every reason to suppose they will, we have to expect that, within six or seven years, it would require, to pay off the debt then existing, more money than there is in the world, or more goods than can be produced in one year by all of the major countries in the Western World.

The international debt defaults of the year 1931 and their aftermath were contemporaneously described as a 'world economic collapse'. Today there are widespread fears of a new collapse this time involving sums of money fifty to one hundred times greater than in 1931, managed by a banking system infinitely more interdependent and complex than could have been imagined just a few years ago.

The Incredible Eurodollar is a prophetic book. Written largely between 1978 and 1980 it accurately forecasts the alarms beginning in 1982. Professors Hogan and Pearce make it clear that world authorities should not be considering how best to support the present system. They should be considering instead how best to end it with a minimum of fuss. What is called for is a new look, not just at present difficulties, but at the whole of our monetary institutions including money itself.

RASTAMAN

The Rastafarian Movement in England

Ernest Cashmore

Since the mid-1970s when the Rastafarian movement first appeared on the streets of England, its presence has provoked suspicion and anxiety. The sight of bizarre-looking black youths, their hair coiled into 'dreadlocks', carrying makeshift prayersticks and preaching the divinity of Haile Selassie, has aroused consternation, resentment, and often outright hostility. Yet this is a movement which has brought an exhilarating and positive new force into the lives of thousands of young blacks and for this reason alone it constitutes the most important development in the history of the West Indian presence in England.

In *Rastaman* Ernest Cashmore has succeeded for the first time in penetrating the mystique of this exclusive movement, whose policy of total non-contact with whites has proved to date such an obstacle to an understanding of it. Cashmore first provides a careful and richly-documented analysis of the genesis and development of the movement, then investigates the effects of external reactions to it and, in particular, explores what kind of subjective meaning the movement has for its members. Cashmore takes the story from sixteenth-century Jamaica and the roots of the movement there, to the streets of present-day Handsworth and Brixton; from the Rastas' puzzling relationship with their reluctant prophet Marcus Garvey, to their intriguing liaison with the punk rock movement and the popular music industry.

Rastaman is the result of two years of patient research and field work, during which time Cashmore was able to move freely among the Rastas themselves and to ask them about their feelings, commitments and ambitions. It provides a unique insight into the nature of the movement in England and into the blacks' own view of their position in modern society.

The Incredible Eurodollar
  W. P. Hogan and I. F. Pearce   £2.95 ☐
Rastaman *Ernest Cashmore*   £2.95 ☐
Socialism in a Cold Climate
  Edited by John Griffith   £2.95 ☐

*All these books are available at your local
bookshop or newsagent, or can be ordered
direct by post. Just tick the titles you want and
fill in the form below.*

———————————————————————————

Name ....

Address..

      ....

      ....

Write to Unwin Cash Sales, PO Box 11,
Falmouth, Cornwall TR10 9EN.

Please enclose remittance to the value of the
cover price plus:

UK: 45p for the first book plus 20p for the
second book, thereafter 14p for each
additional book ordered, to a maximum
charge of £1.63.

BFPO and EIRE: 45p for the first book plus
20p for the second book and 14p for the next 7
books and thereafter 8p per book.

OVERSEAS: 75p for the first book plus 21p
per copy for each additional book.

Unwin Paperbacks reserve the right to show
new retail prices on covers, which may differ
from those previously advertised in the text or
elsewhere. Postage rates are also subject to
revision.